Unstoppable Me

A Type 1 Diabetes Guide and Journey Book for Young Adults, Tweens, and Anyone In Between

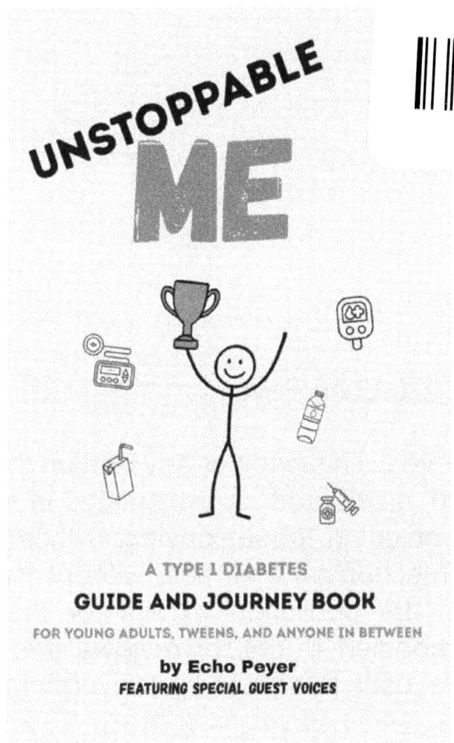

written by: Echo Peyer

with Special Guests:
Courtney Cotton Dobbins
Matti Anderson
Leah Vasquez
Tavia Vital, BSN, BA, RN, CDCES

ISBN: 979-8-9985419-5-7

First printing, 2026.
Missfit Press
Colorado Springs, CO
www.missfitpress.com

DEDICATION

Mom! Dad! Siblings! Niblings! Family and Friends! – for supporting smiling through every crazy thing I do. You are my village, my rock, my crew. Hayden and Kennedy – for showing patience every single day, especially the ones when I really didn't know what to do…I am here because of you.

This Guide and Journey Book Belongs To:

Table of Contents

Introduction: Welcome to the Club You Didn't Ask to Join

Hello you! Congratulations! You're now a card-carrying member of the Type 1 Diabetes Club. Didn't sign up? Well, neither did any of us. But here we are, navigating life with insulin pumps, counting carbohydrates like it's a competitive sport, and sometimes questioning our pancreas with, "What exactly is your job?"

Welcome to *Unstoppable Me: A Type 1 Diabetes Guide & Journey Book*

First things first: this book is **not** here to guilt-trip you, pressure you, or convince you that you need to become some kind of perfect Diabetes Ninja Warrior. This is a guide, a pep talk, and a toolbox for living your best life with Type 1—**messy days, weird blood sugars, mistakes, victories, and everything in between.**

A Note About Me

I'm not a physician or a Certified Diabetes Care and Education Specialist (though I did start training for that once!). What I *am* is a fellow T1D buddy who's been doing this for 38 years. I've learned by being confused, messing up, pivoting, and eventually figuring things out. I also spent ten years working in a nationally known endocrinology clinic, which taught me more about myself—and diabetes—than any job ever could.

Most of what you'll read here is medically solid (thanks Tavia!), but everything is rooted in lived experience—mine and the experiences of other people with Type 1. We're everywhere. You've probably spotted another T1D "in the wild" without even realizing it.

Why You're Here

Maybe someone gave you this book. Maybe you found it on your own. Maybe your great-aunt—the one who buys you sugar-free chocolate bunnies every spring—slipped it into your backpack. However, it landed in your hands, I'm glad it did.

This book covers only one part of my life: the part where I have Type 1 Diabetes. I'm a whole person, and so are you. Diabetes is part of our story, but it's not the whole thing. You'll relate to some of what I share, and some of it won't match your experience at all—and that's exactly how it should be. **My truth is mine. Your truth is yours.**

What This Journey Really Looks Like

Life with T1D can be exhausting, scary, annoying, boring, hilarious, unpredictable, and downright ridiculous. Sometimes all in the same day. It's a constant, ever-changing adventure that asks a lot from us—but it also teaches us things most people never learn.

As you read, think about what *you* would add to the list of what diabetes feels like. What words would you use?

____

____

____

____

Here's what we're going to do:

•**Laugh:** Because diabetes gives us plenty of absurd situations (like dropping your juice box in public and watching others panic like it's a life-or-death emergency).

•**Learn:** We'll break down the technical stuff without boring you to tears.

•**Live:** Pro-tips, real-life advice, and the occasional reminder that your blood sugar does not define your awesomeness.

This book is your roadmap, your friendly nudge, and occasionally your laugh-out-loud distraction when diabetes decides to throw you a curveball (looking at you, 3 a.m. blood sugar alarms). Let's go forth and conquer, shall we? Conquer what, you ask? I'll be honest with you—I'm not exactly sure. Conquer exact carb counts? Ha! Perfect insulin amounts? Ha! Blood sugars consistently hovering around one hundred? Ha ha HA! For now, let's aim to conquer one step at a time. Sound good? Great! Whether you were just diagnosed, or you've been juggling this for years, one thing's for sure: managing diabetes isn't just about insulin and carbs—it's about resilience, humor, and remembering that being human is a messy, wonderful thing.

You are more than your numbers, your charts, or your diagnosis. You're YOU – and that's your strength. You are Unstoppable.

From the People Who Get It

If you've ever tried to explain T1D to someone and watched their eyes glaze over somewhere between "basal rate" and "no, I can't just not eat carbs," you already know this: there's nothing like hearing from people who *actually live it*.

So, throughout this journey, you'll be introduced to a few fellow T1Ds who know the highs, the lows, the rage boluses, the "why is my pump beeping in the middle of Target," and the weirdly specific joy of a perfect arrow.

These aren't polished, inspirational, "my diagnosis made me a superhero" stories. These are real humans talking about real moments—funny ones, messy ones, triumphant ones, and the ones that make you want to throw your glucometer across the room. They're here because they're honest, they're generous, and they're willing to say the things most people don't.

Think of this section like a group chat you didn't know you needed. The kind where someone says, "Does anyone else…?" and suddenly five people reply, "OMG YES." Welcome to the crew. You're in good company.

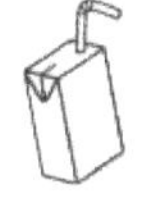

Meet Courtney! Courtney has been living with T1D since the 1970s, which basically makes her our resident legend. She's lived through urine testing, dagger-lancets, early pumps, pump failures, and the rise of tech that actually works. Her story includes her wake-up call: the time she was in a coma with a blood sugar over 1800! She's tough, hilarious, and deeply rooted in the T1D community—especially diabetes camp. When you hear from Courtney, you're getting the kind of wisdom that only comes from five decades of figuring this out in real time.

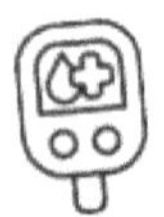

Say hello to Matti! Matti was diagnosed four years ago at age eleven and is now a competitive dancer who manages T1D with the same determination she brings to the stage. She's learned early that diabetes is part science, part intuition, and part "trust your body even when your tech is being dramatic." She's a Youth Advocate, a big sister to two sweet little sisters, and someone who's already using her voice to help other teens feel less alone. From Matti you can expect practical tips, real talk, and the kind of encouragement only another teen T1D can give.

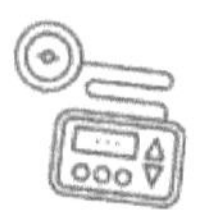

Please meet Leah! Leah found out she had T1D at age 10 in the middle of a medical whirlwind—appendix burst, emergency surgery, the whole thing. She's learned the hard way that diabetes takes a team, not a solo act, and she's big on honesty, humor, and asking for help before burnout hits. She's active, faith-centered, and full of practical hacks for sports, cold weather, and surviving the "Can you have that?" questions. When learning from Leah you know you are getting grounded, heartfelt advice from someone who's been through a lot and still shows up with strength.

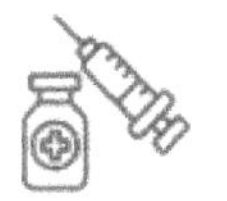

This is Tavia! Tavia Vital, BSN, BA, RN, CDCES, has been living with T1D since she was two years old—back in the days of urine strips cut into thirds, giant needles, and glucose meters the size of lunchboxes. She grew up learning to advocate for herself long before CGMs, pumps, or smartphones existed. Not only is she our Unstoppable Me medical editor, she is also the Director of Intensive Diabetes Management at Integrated Diabetes Services LLC. Tavia shares her blends lived experience, clinical expertise, and a whole lot of heart to help people with T1D feel capable, confident, and never alone.

Meet Betty

A story about the monster you didn't ask for... and the one you learn to live with.

A long time ago—which somehow doesn't feel that long ago—I realized my diabetes wasn't going anywhere. It was here.

Forever.

Forever ever?

Yep. Forever.

It was something different inside my body, different from my parents, my siblings, my friends. Different from who I was before. But even though it was with me to stay, it wasn't here to change *who* I was. Or *why* I was. Or *how* I was. It was simply... here.

Like a pet.

Not a pet I would've asked for. Heck no.

An annoying pet.

A greedy pet.

A make-me-different-from-almost-everyone-else kind of pet.

A terrible, horrible, no-good, very-bad pet.

A *monster* of a pet.

That was it.

A monster.

A Pet Monster.

I had been given a pet monster, and I had no earthly choice but to take care of it.

So I did.

Grudgingly.

Sparingly.

With as little attention as possible.

I hid It from new people. Minimized It with people who already knew me. I remember winning movie tickets in middle school and sitting next to one of the cutest boys in 8th grade. Halfway through the movie, he got up to use the restroom. My best friend instantly became the lookout while I pulled out my syringe and glass vial to draw up a few overdue units. (How many carbs are in movie popcorn and candy? Let's not ruin the mood by calculating.)

I dosed quickly, tucked everything away, and felt relieved for two reasons:

1. I'd finally taken the insulin I needed.
2. I'd hidden it from someone I thought might judge me.

So, I kept my pet monster quiet. Behind the scenes. Ignored. But here's the thing about monsters: they don't like being ignored.

Mine bucked. It clawed. It demanded attention. And eventually, it revolted. It screamed, pushed, kicked, knocked me flat, and landed me in the hospital—surrounded by tubes, beeping machines, and well-meaning lectures about the importance of paying attention to my pet monster every minute of every day.

I was furious.

I wanted to scream, *NO. I'm done. I don't want to do this anymore.*

But I didn't scream.

Because I wasn't done.

Not really.

I didn't let my pet monster take over on purpose. I just didn't want It to exist. I didn't want the responsibility, the embarrassment, the sideways looks in restaurant bathrooms while I took my shot.

So I did the only thing I could do if I wanted to stay alive.

I accepted my pet monster.

I named It.

Betty. Clever, right?!

Betty was part of me—permanently and forever more.

Forever ever.

For EVER ever?

Yep.

I didn't want a pet monster, but I finally understood that Betty and I were going to have to figure out how to live together. In harmony. In peace. In as much balance as we could muster, moment by moment.

It was time for Betty and me to get… organized.

PRO TIP: Since this is a guide and journey, here's your first piece of guidance from someone who's been there: Accept your Betty. Or your Spike. Or your Mellie (short for "mellitus" ha). Your Very Own Pet Monster.

It needs attention. Food. Medicine. Water. Rest.

If you can organize your life enough to support your pet monster, it will mostly stay calm, usually stay out of the limelight, and—for the most part—let you live the life you want.

Let your Betty be a partner, not an enemy.

ACTIVITY: Your Pet Monster

Name your pet monster. Say hello. Introduce yourself to them here and let them know what your expectations of them are. Remember, you can't choose to send them on their way – but you can choose to keep them organized:

Okay it's time to get really creative! Use this space to draw your pet monster:

Diabetes 101 –The Basics Without the Boredom

So, what exactly is Type 1 Diabetes? Imagine this: your pancreas is like that one coworker who quietly kept things running in the background. Then one day, they walked out of the office, slammed the door, and left you a sticky note that says, "You're in charge now."

Welcome to your new job: Full-Time Pancreas Manager. The good news? You've got insulin, blood sugar meters, and some pretty sweet technology to help you out. The bad news? There's no off-the-clock time.

But don't worry, we'll break it down, so it doesn't feel like you're drowning in medical jargon.

What Happened to My Pancreas?

Let's start with the basics. Type 1 Diabetes (T1D) happens when your immune system goes rogue and attacks the beta cells in your pancreas. These cells were in charge of making insulin, which is like the body's Uber for glucose. Without insulin, glucose (sugar from food) just wanders around your bloodstream like a tourist without Google Maps.

No insulin = no energy = you feel like a zombie.

But here's where you step in. With synthetic insulin (shoutout to modern medicine!), you take charge, delivering insulin yourself through shots, pens, or pumps. It's teamwork… kind of.

The Jargon Cheat Sheet

You'll hear a lot of terms thrown around at doctor appointments. Here's a cheat sheet:

- **Blood Sugar (Glucose):** The sugar in your blood that your body uses for energy. Too much? Hyperglycemia. Too little? Hypoglycemia.
- **Insulin:** A hormone that is like a magic key that lets sugar into your cells. Without enough of it, the sugar starts to look like a long line waiting to get into a concert. Insulin is the VIP Pass, without it no one gets in, even if they have tickets!
- **Basal vs. Bolus:**
- Basal is your all-day all-night insulin (like background music).
- Bolus is your food insulin and your high glucose correction insulin (the opening acts and the cleanup crews)
- **A1C:** A fancy name of a blood test that tells you your average blood sugar over the last three months. Think of it as your diabetes GPA.

It's Not Your Fault (Seriously)

Let's clear this up right now:

- You didn't get T1D because you ate too much sugar.

- It's not something you could've prevented.
- And no, kale smoothies with cinnamon won't "cure" it. Neither will weight loss, non-stop exercise, or okra tea!

Your immune system just decided to go all ninja on your pancreas. That's it. It's nobody's fault, especially not yours.

Why Is Managing T1D So Weird?

Here's the deal: Type 1 Diabetes doesn't play by the rules.

- You can eat the exact same breakfast two days in a row and get completely different blood sugar readings.
- Stress, exercise, sleep, and even the weather can mess with your numbers.
- Sometimes, it feels like your body is trying to prank you.

That's because diabetes management is more of an art than a science. It's not about being "perfect" (spoiler: no one is). It's about figuring out what works for you most of the time.

PRO TIP: The First Rule of Diabetes Club

If you're feeling overwhelmed, that's normal. Learning to manage T1D is like learning a new language while juggling flaming torches. Start small, ask questions, and remind yourself: you're not alone.

And hey, if all else fails, just blame your pancreas.

ACTIVITY: Come on, let's be real! What's something that you find completely WEIRD about your T1D?

A Day in the Life – The Real Deal

Managing Type 1 Diabetes isn't just a "sometimes" thing—it's an all-day, every-day, no-vacation kind of deal. But don't worry, you'll get the hang of it. Let's take a walk through a typical day in the life of someone managing T1D, with all the highs (literally) and lows (also literally).

Morning: Wake Up and Check In

Your alarm goes off. But before you roll out of bed, you grab your meter or glance at your Continuous Glucose Monitor (CGM) to see how the night treated you.

- **High?** Maybe that late-night snack caught up to you. Time for some insulin, a glass of water, and a deep sigh.
- **Low?** Time to chug some juice like a toddler at snack time. Just kidding. You might be surprised how little it sometimes takes to get your glucose back safely in the morning!
- **Just Right?** Congrats, Goldilocks. This is your moment to shine.

PRO TIP: Your morning blood sugar can feel like it will make or break your day. Starting out Just Right will give you flexibility and freedom throughout the rest of the day – an in-range blood sugar is easier to keep steady than correcting an out of range one!

Breakfast: The Carb Conundrum

Ah, breakfast—the most math-filled meal of the day. Here's where you do some quick calculations:

1. How many carbs are in your cereal, toast, or smoothie?
2. How much insulin do you need to cover it?
3. Will your blood sugar behave, or is it planning a surprise rollercoaster?

PRO TIP: Always keep backup snacks nearby after eating large amounts of carbs. Pancakes and cereal are delicious, but they don't always play nicely with your blood sugar.

School/Work: Juggling Act

Managing diabetes during the day can feel like you're secretly running a side hustle while also trying to focus on algebra, meetings, or TikTok trends.

- **The CGM Alarm:** The unmistakable BEEP BEEP that tells everyone, "Yes, I have a medical condition, and no, it's not a big deal unless I pass out."
- **Snack Stash:** Granola bars, juice boxes, and glucose tabs become your best friends.
- **Explaining to Others:**
  "No, I can't 'just try keto.'"
  "Yes, I can eat that donut. I just need insulin first."

Lunch: The Guessing Game Continues

Lunchtime often comes with challenges like mystery carbs in cafeteria food or peer pressure to order fries.

- The key? Balance. Take your insulin, eat what you love, and don't overthink every bite.
- Also, pack a lunch if you can. It's easier to manage when you know what's in it.

Afternoon: The Energy Dip

Blood sugar highs and lows love to mess with your focus. If you're feeling:

- **Foggy or Shaky:** You might be going low. Confirm it, treat it fast, and keep moving.
- **Tired or Cranky:** A high might be dragging you down. If it is, drink water, take insulin, and remind yourself that it's only a bad moment, not a bad day.

Exercise: The Wild Card

Working out with T1D is like playing tag with your blood sugar—it might chase you down, or you might outrun it.

- **Plan ahead:** Check your blood sugar before you start.
- **During:** Keep snacks or glucose tabs on hand in case you go low.

- **After:** Watch for delayed lows (the "gotcha" moment your body loves to pull hours after a workout).

Dinner: Another Round of Carb Math

Dinner can be tricky, especially if you're eating out or trying something new.

- Apps like MyFitnessPal or your favorite Ai program can help with carb counts.
- Another pro tip: Enjoy your food! Don't let the numbers take all the fun out of eating.

Nighttime: The Final Check-In

Before you hit the hay, it's time for one last blood sugar check.

- **High?** Adjust with insulin.
- **Low?** Snack time! Keep it light so you don't wake up high.
- Set alarms if you're worried about overnight lows or use your CGM to monitor.

The Not-So-Perfect Days

Some days, no matter how much you plan, things just don't go right.

- That's okay. Diabetes doesn't follow the rules, and you're allowed to feel frustrated.
- Remember: You're doing your best.

PRO TIP: Laugh When You Can

Diabetes is serious, but life doesn't have to be. Find the humor in the little things—like when your CGM picks the loudest moment possible to alert you, or when a well-meaning stranger asks if you've 'tried cinnamon'!

ACTIVITY: Think of the silliest question someone has asked you about diabetes. Can you think of a good way to reply the next time someone asks you something similar?

____

____

____

____

____

____

____

____

____

____

____

____

____

____

____

Tools of the Trade – Gearing Up for the Journey

Managing Type 1 Diabetes isn't a solo act—it's more like a one-person band. You've got gadgets, gizmos, and the occasional snack stash that would make a scout proud. Let's break down the tools that will help you live your best life (and maybe make you feel a little like a cyborg in the process).

1. The MVP: Insulin

Insulin is your lifesaver, plain and simple. It comes in a few forms, and you get to pick the one that suits your lifestyle:

- **Pens:** Discreet, portable, and perfect for quick doses. Plus, they make you feel like a diabetes ninja.
- **Syringes:** Old school but reliable. Think of it as the classic flip phone of diabetes management.
- **Pumps:** Fancy little devices that deliver insulin through a tiny tube under your skin. They're like having a personal assistant for your pancreas.

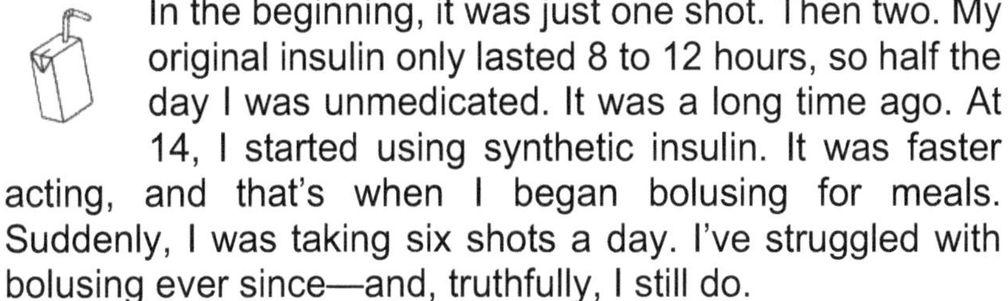

In the beginning, it was just one shot. Then two. My original insulin only lasted 8 to 12 hours, so half the day I was unmedicated. It was a long time ago. At 14, I started using synthetic insulin. It was faster acting, and that's when I began bolusing for meals. Suddenly, I was taking six shots a day. I've struggled with bolusing ever since—and, truthfully, I still do.

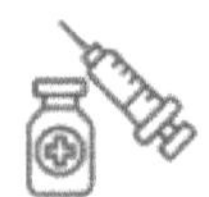

I started on animal insulin—first cow, then pork. The needles were thick and long, and the injections left my thighs hard and scarred. Eventually, synthetic insulins and smaller needles changed everything.

2. Blood Sugar Monitoring: Eyes on the Prize

Keeping tabs on your blood sugar is like checking the weather, it helps you decide what to do next.

- **Meters:** The OG tool. Prick your finger, get a drop of blood, and voilà—instant blood sugar reading.
- **Continuous Glucose Monitors (CGMs):** These are game changers. They track your blood sugar all day and night, sending data to your phone or device. (Bonus: You'll feel like a tech wizard when you show someone the graph of your glucose trends.) (See section *Diabetes Tech* for more info on CGMs)

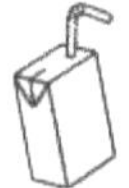

At 13, I got my first glucometer. It took two whole minutes to give me a result—forever, right? I ditched it for two months. Those lancets were like daggers. I wasn't compliant.

Back then, we didn't check blood sugar with a meter. We tested urine. That gave us sugar levels from 6 to 8 hours earlier. It always ran high. And yes, I wet the bed a lot. Don't be ashamed if this happens—it happens to all of us, at all ages.

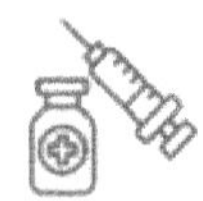

When I was young, families were sent home with urine tests because people believed finger pokes were too painful for young kids. My parents pushed for blood glucose strips and a lancet device nicknamed “The Guillotine.” The strips were expensive and not covered by insurance, so they cut them into halves and thirds. You matched the color on the strip to the vial: 20, 40, 80, 120, 180, 240, 400, 800. Results took minutes. When glucose meters became available, my parents paid out of pocket. They were huge and required multiple steps.

3. Low Supplies: Your First Aid Kit

Lows happen, and when they do, you need to be ready. Stock up on:

- Juice boxes (the kid-sized ones fit perfectly in a bag).
- Glucose tablets or Smarties (chalky but effective).
- Candy (Skittles are a favorite for a reason).
- Crackers or granola bars for the follow-up snack.
- Glucose (Dextrose) gel (extra super-fast absorption).
- Glucagon (important to have on hand just in case a severe low glucose happens).

PRO TIP: Store some of these items next to your bed, in your diabetes bag, in your locker, your backpack, in your desk or locker at work. Have backups for your backups for low treatments!

4. High Supplies: The Cleanup Crew

Dealing with a high blood sugar? Time to break out the hydration and insulin correction tools:

- **Water:** The unsung hero of blood sugar highs. It helps flush out extra sugar.
- **Ketone Strips:** If you're feeling sick, these help you check for ketones (the not-so-fun sidekick of high blood sugar).
- **Troubleshooting Hyperglycemia Plan:** It includes an insulin dosing plan, of how often to check your blood glucose or look at your CGM, how often to check for ketones, and when to call your Diabetes Healthcare Team if your glucose keeps staying too high or is too high too frequently.

5. Apps and Tech: Your Digital Sidekicks

There's an app for almost everything, and diabetes management is no exception.

- **Carb Counting Apps:** MyFitnessPal, CalorieKing, or Cronometer help you figure out how many carbs are in your meal.
- **Diabetes Management Apps:** Apps like Dexcom, LibreLink, Tidepool, or SugarMate sync with CGMs for easy tracking.
- **Logbooks:** Yes, old-school pen-and-paper works too, but apps make it easier to spot trends.

6. Emergency Gear: Be Prepared for Anything

Life is unpredictable, but you don't have to be. Pack a kit with:

- Extra insulin and supplies (pens, syringes, pump reservoirs).
- Batteries or a charger for your devices.
- A glucagon kit for severe lows (make sure someone you trust knows how to use it).
- An "In Case of Emergency" card with your info, so people know you have T1D.

PRO TIP: Wear a medical ID that states: Insulin Dependent Diabetes. Not all emergency responders can look inside a wallet to find an In Case of Emergency Card. Don't worry...there are a lot of different styles of medical ID to select from online. It can look just like a watch band or jewelry if you prefer.

7. Snacks: The Unsung Hero

Let's be real—diabetes snacks aren't just for emergencies. They're also for life's little hiccups.

Keep a stash of:

- Trail mix (customizable and delicious).
- Popcorn (light on the carbs but satisfying).
- Nut butter packets (portable and filling).

8. Support Squad: You Don't Have to Go It Alone

Your most valuable "tool" isn't a gadget—it's your support system.

- **Friends and Family:** Teach them the basics so they can help when you need it.
- **Healthcare Team:** Endocrinologists, diabetes educators, and nutritionists are your go-to pros.
- **Online Communities:** Join groups, forums, or social media pages where people get it.

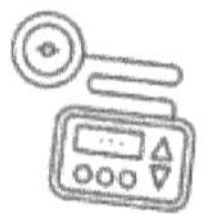

I would recommend keeping at least one extra set of supplies (pump sets, syringes, CGM, etc.) in your bag. I have one in my Basketball ~ Volleyball ~ Whatever-Sport-I'm-Doing-Bag, one in my suitcase, and one in my diabetes bag. My diabetes bag is a small bag I carry around with me everywhere. It has things for lows, extra pump sights, my nasal spray, and my finger prick set (in case my CGM is inaccurate which it will be sometimes).

PRO TIP: Always carry extra supplies because the universe loves to throw curveballs at the worst times.

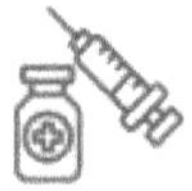

EXTRA PRO TIP: If you are realizing that your supplies kit or plan is missing something, take time now to jot down what you need to get:

____

____

____

ACTIVITY: Customize Your Kit

Diabetes is personal, so your toolkit should be too. Experiment with what works best for your routine, lifestyle, and preferences. And don't be afraid to upgrade your gear when new tech comes out! Try different bags or carrying kits to see what works for you. Also: stickers, patches and pump/cgm covers can help you share your personal STYLE.

One last word: Bejeweled

Diabetes Tech – Mastering the Tools of T1D Tech

Welcome to the exciting world of diabetes technology! Whether you're a tech-savvy pro who can troubleshoot a CGM in your sleep, or someone curious about what all the gadgets can do, this chapter is for you.

Some of this might already be common knowledge, but there's always something new to learn—or a fresh way to think about how tech can simplify your T1D life. From continuous glucose monitors (CGMs) to insulin pumps, we'll explore how these tools work, their pros and cons, and tips for getting the most out of them.

Let's dive into the tech that's changing the game for people with T1D.

1. Continuous Glucose Monitors (CGMs)

CGMs are the unsung heroes of diabetes tech, giving you a near-constant stream of blood sugar data without the need for endless finger sticks.

How CGMs Work:

- A tiny sensor sits just under your skin, measuring glucose levels in your interstitial fluid (the fluid around your cells).
- Data is sent to a receiver, smartphone app, or smartwatch, giving you updates every 1-5 minutes.

- Most CGMs can alert you to highs, lows, and rapid changes in blood sugar.
- A CGM can be used with multiple daily injections of insulin or as part of a hybrid, automated insulin delivery (pump) system.

Popular CGM Brands:

- **Dexcom:** Loved for its accuracy and smartphone connectivity. Pairs with several automated insulin delivery systems (pumps).
- **Freestyle Libre:** Known for its simplicity lower price tag. Pairs with several automated insulin delivery systems (pumps).
- **Medtronic:** Guardian or Simplera Sync. Pair with Medtronic pumps or a smartpen called InPen.

Tips for CGM Success:

- **Calibrate (if needed):** Some CGMs require periodic calibrations with finger sticks for accuracy.
- **Use Alerts Wisely:** Customize your high and low alerts to avoid alarm fatigue.
- **Look for Trends:** Use your data to spot patterns, not just react to individual numbers.

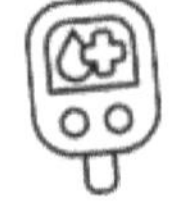

Through my journey, I've learned that managing Type 1 Diabetes is about more than numbers. It's about balance, patience, and learning to trust myself. I've learned practical strategies that help me stay in range, like setting timers so I don't forget to eat, drinking extra water when my blood sugar is high, and being careful not to stack insulin and cause dangerous lows. I've also learned that technology, like insulin pumps and continuous glucose monitors, is incredibly helpful...but it's not perfect. If my glucose monitor says I'm fine, but my body feels low, I trust how I feel and check it with a traditional finger poke and meter.

2. Insulin Pumps

Insulin pumps are like having a personal assistant for your diabetes management. They deliver insulin throughout the day, mimicking a functioning pancreas.

How Pumps Work:

- A small device delivers insulin via a thin tube inserted into the skin.
- The small device that holds the insulin (the pump) can be a patch pump (tubeless), or a "tubed" pump.
- You program the pump with your basal rates (background insulin delivery) and boluses (mealtime and correction doses of insulin).

Popular Insulin Pumps:

All popular insulin pump systems today can automate parts of the insulin delivery process. Nearly all require some type of info from you when you plan to eat food, and some adjustment for physical activity.

- **Omnipod 5:** A tubeless, waterproof pump that sticks directly to your skin. Integrated with specific Dexcom and Libre CGMs. Learns an estimated basal rate which adjusts over time based on total daily doses of insulin.

- **Tandem t:slim X2 and Tandem Mobi:** Features advanced algorithms, options for alternative setting profiles, and integration with specific Dexcom and Libre CGMs.
- **Medtronic MiniMed:** Features a strong algorithm which uses total daily dose to learn basal and correction needs over time.
- **Twiist:** Originally developed and made available in 2024 by the Open-Source Community (to learn something amazing, Google #WeAreNotWaiting). Pairs with certain Libre sensors and the Eversense 365 sensor.
- **iLet:** Features a non-specific carb dosing method of "announcing" meals. Users select the options of normal, less, or more than normal sized meals and the system learns over time the average dose needed by meal size and by type of meal.
- **Open Source Systems: Loop, Trio, or Android APS:** Uses FDA approved devices (pumps, sensors) with non-FDA approved algorithms in a cellphone app. Each system offers robust features that are not available in commercial systems. (Think: Master Ninja Level Insulin Pump Systems)

Tips for Pumping Success:

- **Site Rotation:** Change infusion sites regularly to avoid scar tissue.

- **Bolus Timing:** Pre-bolus (deliver insulin 15-20 minutes before normal meals) to stay ahead of blood sugar spikes.
- **Backup Plan:** Always have syringes or pens as a backup in case of pump failure. Keep a note or file on your phone with instructions on how to calculate your doses for a backup injection plan.
- **Patterns:** Learn about identifying patterns. Patterns are key to getting useful insulin dose adjustments and setting up strategies for hard to dose for foods, or for different types of physical activity, or other glucose challenges.

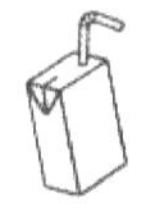

In my mid-40s, my pump failed. I thought it was food poisoning—I couldn't stop vomiting. My blood sugar was high. I changed my infusion site and took extra insulin. Still high. Still sick. I prayed to live. I started manual injections and went to the ER. Four days in the hospital. I never thought my pump would fail. Please—be ready.

If I were to share only one **PRO TIP** with you it's this one:

Pumps fail. Always keep long-acting insulin at home. Know your carb ratio—how many carbs per unit of insulin? If your blood sugar is high, how many units do you need to bring it down? (Blood sugar - 100) ÷ your correction factor. This calculation is different for everyone. Know how many units of long-acting insulin you need today. <u>This is life-saving information</u>.

3. Smart Pens and Hybrid Approaches

Not ready for a pump? Smart insulin pens offer a great middle ground. They track your doses and help with timing, giving you some of the benefits of pump technology without the commitment.

Popular Smart Pens:

- **InPen:** Tracks doses, offers reminders, and syncs with an app to calculate your doses and help you analyze your data.

4. Closed-Loop Systems

Sometimes called an “artificial pancreas,” “hybrid-closed-loop”, or “closed-loop” system, they connect CGMs and pumps to automatically adjust insulin delivery based on your glucose levels and some input by the wearer of the pump and sensor.

How They Work:

- The CGM sends data to the pump.
- The pump adjusts basal rates and/or delivers micro-boluses to keep blood sugar in range.
- Every system has its own unique pros and cons.

Who Should Consider Closed-Loop?

- People who want tighter control with less effort.
- Those who experience frequent highs or lows.

- Hybrid-closed-loop systems are considered the gold standard plan for people who require insulin dosing to live (that would be US!)

5. Diabetes Apps and Data Management

Your phone can be your best diabetes sidekick. With the right apps, you can track data, spot trends, and make more informed decisions.

Must-Try Apps for T1D:

- **MySugr:** Tracks everything from blood sugars to carbs and insulin. Bonus: It's playful and fun.
- **Glooko:** Syncs data from multiple devices for a complete overview.
- **Tidepool:** Syncs data from multiple devices for a complete overview. Has a customizable note taking cell-phone app and well-designed reports for reviewing data trends with your notes.
- **Sugarmate:** Adds customizable alerts and integration with CGMs.
- **SNAQ:** Take a photo of your food. SNAQ uses AI to list the meal's ingredients and nutrients, including carb counts. It acts as a pictorial log you can use when reviewing your data trends (patterns)

6. Wearable Tech for Exercise and Lifestyle

Devices like Fitbit, Garmin, Oura Ring, and Apple Watch can monitor your workouts, heart rate, and even blood sugar (if synced with a CGM).

Lifestyle Hacks:

- Use reminders to check blood sugar during workouts and to adjust your insulin before your workouts (if needed).
- Track how exercise impacts your trends over time.

7. Challenges of Diabetes Tech

No tech is perfect, and T1D gadgets come with their own set of frustrations.

Common Issues:

- **Sensor Failures and Temporary Issues:** CGMs can occasionally stop working, especially in extreme temperatures or after intense workouts. The sensor can be inaccurate. It might stop giving your readings for awhile, then start working again. Give it some time and **MAKE SURE YOU ARE DRINKING YOU WATER!!** Dehydration can cause CGM readings to jump around. Also, breath. Stress can cause your numbers to go high.
- **Device Costs:** Tech isn't cheap. Make sure to explore insurance coverage or manufacturer programs for assistance.

- **Learning Curve:** Getting comfortable with new devices takes time, so be patient with yourself.

8. Staying Up to Date

Diabetes tech evolves quickly, so staying informed is key.

How to Keep Up:

- Follow T1D forums and social media accounts for the latest updates.
- Ask your Endocrinologist and your Diabetes Care and Education Specialist about new devices or upgrades.
- Attend diabetes conferences or webinars to see what's on the horizon.

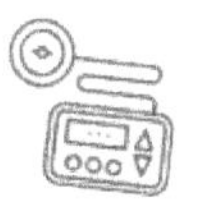

PRO TIP: While tech makes life with T1D easier, remember that you are the ultimate decision-maker. Devices provide tools and data, but your intuition and experience are equally important. Trust yourself, you're doing amazing.

ACTIVITY: Note any of the topics above that you want to learn more about. Share this list with your clinical care team – they can help answer your questions and share options for you to consider.

____

____

____

____

____

Highs, Lows, and Everything In Between – Handling the Ups and Downs

If diabetes were a movie, blood sugar levels would be the unpredictable plot twists: the highs that leave you feeling sluggish, the lows that make you shaky, and the rare perfect number that feels like winning the lottery. Let's talk about how to navigate these moments without losing your mind—or your sense of humor.

The Highs (Hyperglycemia): When Your Blood Sugar Won't Chill

A high blood sugar (hyperglycemia) happens when there's too much sugar in your blood and not enough insulin to handle it. Symptoms include:

- Feeling tired or sluggish, like you've been hit by a nap truck.
- Dry mouth or extreme thirst (hello, water bottle).
- Frequent bathroom trips (because you're drinking all that water).

Common Causes of Highs:

- Forgot to take insulin (oops—it happens).
- Skipped the pre-bolus (oops—it happens).
- Ate more carbs than expected (because fries are sneaky).

- Stress, illness, or hormones deciding to mess with you.

How to Handle It:

1. **Check Your Blood Sugar:** Confirm it's high before taking action.
2. **Correct With Insulin:** Use your pump, pen, or syringe to bring it down. Follow your Healthcare Provider's recommendations.
3. **Drink Water:** Hydration helps flush out the extra sugar.
4. **Check for Ketones:** If you're over 250 mg/dL and feeling unwell, test for ketones. High ketones mean it's time to call your doctor.

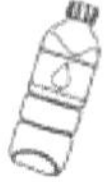

Highs happen to everyone. Don't beat yourself up over it, just take action, rest as you can, and move on.

The Lows (Hypoglycemia): When You Need Sugar, Stat

A low blood sugar (hypoglycemia) happens when there's too much insulin and not enough glucose in your system. Symptoms include:

- Feeling shaky, weak, or lightheaded.
- Sweating like you just ran a marathon (even if you didn't move).
- Feeling irritable or confused (sometimes you'll even snap at people and not realize it).

Common Causes of Lows:

- Took too much insulin (math is hard, okay?).
- Missed a meal or snack after taking a dose of fast acting insulin (so much to do, so little time!)
- Exercised without enough carbs on board.
- Drinking alcohol (once you are of legal age, of course!). Have an alcohol and diabetes safety plan in place if you decide to drink alcohol.

How to Handle It:

1. **Check Your Blood Sugar:** Anything below 70 mg/dL counts as a low.
2. **Treat It Fast:**

    - Eat or drink 15 grams of fast-acting carbs (juice, candy, glucose tablets).
    - Wait 15 minutes, then check again. If it's still low, repeat.

3. **Follow Up:** Once your blood sugar is stable, you might need to eat a snack to prevent another dip if: you have too much insulin on board, or you were (or will be) physically active.

✓ Many people find the Rule of 15 (eat 15 carbs, recheck blood sugar in 15 minutes) leaves them running too high later. You will learn over time how many carbs your body needs to guide your glucose quickly back to safety without causing a rocket ship pattern after. Don't go with your gut on this one! You may feel like eating everything in sight. This will absolutely lead to super high glucose levels later. Save yourself the frustration.

- ✓ Set yourself up for success. Keep low snacks in every possible place: your bag, locker, car, bedside table, and even that secret pocket in your hoodie. Pre-package a normal amount of low glucose treatments. Carry several pre-packaged treatments, just in case.

- ✓ **ONE MORE IMPORTANT NOTE ON LOWS!**
    - Step 1: learn about glucagon if you haven't yet. It is an emergency low glucose treatment. It can be lifesaving.
    - Step 2: teach those closest to you (at home, at school, at work) how to administer glucagon if you haven't yet. I repeat: it can be lifesaving!!

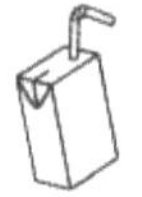

I'll never forget Halloween night, 1977. We got to go outside our neighborhood, and my bag was full of candy. That night, I passed out with candy all around me. My parents rushed me to the ER. They had no idea how much I'd eaten—but I had NOT overdone it with my candy. It was a low blood sugar. Best Halloween ever ha!

The Rollercoaster: When Highs and Lows Tag-Team You

Sometimes your blood sugar can feel like it's auditioning for a theme park ride. One minute you're low, the next you're high, and you're left wondering if you'll ever level out.

How to Handle It:

- **Stay Calm:** It's frustrating, but it's temporary.
- **Focus on the Cause:** Was it a meal, stress, or just a random diabetes moment?
- **Adjust Gradually:** Avoid overcorrecting (e.g., don't treat a low with an entire pizza, tempting as it is).

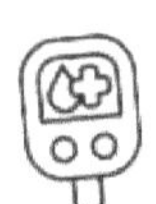

Avoid 'stacking' insulin. This is when you take insulin to cover carbs, then take more insulin to cover more carbs. Then want to snack some more so you take MORE insulin to cover MORE carbs! Too much insulin to fast can cause a severe low.

REMINDER: YOU ARE Not a Number

Your blood sugar is just one part of who you are, it's data that helps you determine your next step. It doesn't define your worth, your abilities, or your awesomeness. When things get tough, remind yourself:

- Everyone with diabetes has ups and downs.
- No one gets it "perfect" all the time.
- You're doing the best you can, and that's enough.

When to Call for Backup

Sometimes diabetes pulls a fast one, and you need help. Call your doctor or diabetes team if:

- Your blood sugar is consistently above 250 mg/dL or below 70 mg/dL, and you can't fix it.
- You're feeling sick and can't keep food or water down.
- You're just overwhelmed and need guidance (because that's what they're there for).

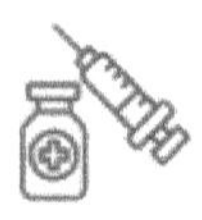

PRO TIP: Some influencers on social media call themselves 'flatliners'. They use AI to create fake glucose graphs. Don't compare your diabetes to someone else! Even the real flatter glucose graph online gurus have whacky numbers sometimes.

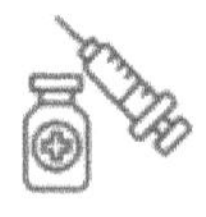

ACTIVITY: Do you have your low glucose treatment items stocked and ready to go? If not, make a list of what you need. What's your favorite? Fruit snacks! Apple juice! Smarties! Skittles! When you're stocked, here is a cHalLeNgE! Set a time and see how fast you can grab a low treatment from everywhere in your home. Where are some extra places you should stash some quick-acting carbs?

****

WHEW! Okay, I want to stop and have you take a deep breath.

Another one – slower and deeper. Innnnn and ouuuuut. You have just received a TON of information. Let's check in. Do you need a break? I wouldn't blame you if you did. If fact – let's all stop! Check our blood sugars (at the time of this writing I am riding steady at 165!). Take a stretch. Wiggle your body. Grab a snack. Snuggle your pet. Remember, this is YOUR guide for YOUR journey. Come back when you're ready!

****

Food, Nutrition, and Living Beyond the "Perfect Diet"

Let's be real: food is one of life's greatest joys. It's fuel, it's social, and sometimes, it's just the cure for a bad day. But when you have Type 1 Diabetes, eating comes with some extra planning—and a lot of carb counting. Don't worry, though. You can still enjoy everything from pizza to birthday cake. Let's dig in (pun intended) and talk about eating well with T1D while keeping it realistic, flexible, and enjoyable.

1. Forget the "Perfect Diet."

Spoiler alert: There's no one-size-fits-all diet for people with Type 1 Diabetes. Some folks thrive on low-carb plans, while others rock a more balanced approach. What's most important is finding a way of eating that supports your blood sugar goals, your overall health, and your happiness.

Why Perfection Isn't the Goal:

- **Diabetes Is Dynamic:** What worked yesterday might not work today, and that's okay.
- **Food Is More Than Fuel:** It's culture, celebration, and connection. You don't have to sacrifice that for perfect numbers.

2. Carb Counting Like A Pro (or Close Enough)

Carb counting is like learning a new language. At first, it feels impossible, but with practice, it gets easier. Here's how to level up your carb-counting game:

Start with Labels:

- Food labels are your best friend. Look for "Total Carbohydrate" and adjust for portion size.

Use Tools:

- Apps like MyFitnessPal, Carb Manager, or even simple Google searches can help with carb estimates.
- Weighing food with a kitchen scale can improve accuracy.
- Get some long-handled measuring cup serving spoons. Save time by measuring your food as you scoop and serve it.

Eyeball It:

- You won't always have a scale or measuring cup handy, so practice estimating. (A tennis ball is about 15g of carbs for fruit; a slice of bread is usually around 15g.)

3. Mastering Meals Out

Eating at restaurants can be tricky, but it's totally doable.

Tips for Dining Out:

- **Research the Menu:** Look up carb counts ahead of time if possible.
- **Ask Questions:** Don't hesitate to ask the server about ingredients or portion sizes.
- **Bolus Strategically:** High-fat meals (hello, burgers and fries) may require split dosing or extended boluses.
- **Use your tools:** If the restaurant is not part of a chain, try using an AI app to calculate the carbs using a photo of your meal.

The Dessert Debate:

Yes, you can eat dessert. No, it won't destroy your pancreas—it already called it quits in the insulin making department, remember? Bolus for it, enjoy it, and move on.

4. Snacks That Save the Day

Snacks aren't just for kids. They're your secret weapon against blood sugar chaos when you are physically active, or when you plan to go a long time between meals.

Go-To Low Treatments:

- Glucose tabs (fast and predictable).
- Juice boxes.
- Fruit snacks.

Balanced Snack Ideas:

- Apple slices with peanut butter.
- Cheese sticks and crackers.
- Greek yogurt with a sprinkle of granola.

5. Managing Blood Sugar Rollercoasters

The Infamous Pizza Effect:

High-fat, high-carb meals (like pizza, pasta, and Chinese takeout) digest slowly, causing delayed blood sugar spikes. Sometimes they cause low sugars shortly after the meal, then highs over several hours. I KNOW, seriously?

- **Tip:** Try dual-wave boluses (if you use a pump) or split injections to manage these meals.

The Mysterious Low:

Some meals cause surprise lows (exercise or alcohol often play a role). Keep fast-acting carbs that are made out of dextrose (preferably gel or liquid) nearby to handle these. If your stomach is full of food and your glucose is going low, you need something that can absorb quickly and work its way in and around all the food.

6. Special Diets: Yay or Nay?

From keto to vegan, there are a million diets out there, and you might be tempted to try one. Here's the lowdown:

Low-Carb Diets:

- These can help reduce blood sugar variability, but they're not for everyone.
- Be mindful of the risk of ketones and discuss any drastic changes with your doctor. Your insulin doses may need to be adjusted.

Plant-Based Diets:

- Great for heart health and overall well-being.
- Carb-heavy foods like beans and grains can be tricky to dose for but manageable with practice.

The Best Diet:

The one that works for your body, blood sugar, and lifestyle.

7. When Numbers Get Weird

Sometimes you'll do everything "right" and your blood sugar will still go rogue. Maybe it's the stress, hormones, or the alignment of the planets. Here's what to do when food-related numbers aren't adding up:

- **Pause:** Take a breath. One high or low isn't the end of the world.
- **Adjust:** Correct as needed and move forward.
- **Remember:** You're not a failure—you're a human living with a condition that loves to keep you guessing.

8. Building a Positive Relationship with Food

It's easy to fall into the trap of seeing food as the enemy when you're constantly managing diabetes. But food is your ally—it keeps you going, helps you thrive, and brings joy to your life.

PRO TIP: Food Is Joy

Food is more than numbers—it's culture, celebration, and connection. Don't let diabetes take that away from you. Enjoy your meals, learn as you go, and remind yourself: a high or a low = a learning opportunity!

ACTIVITY: Is there something you've not eaten since your diagnosis because you've been afraid of dosing incorrectly? Let's figure it out now. 1) Write down the food and start researching. Once you've determined the carb count; 2) DOSE AND GO EAT IT! Yummy! Now keep an eye on your levels – check after 30 minutes, 60 minutes, 2 hours and 4 hours. (If you start to feel low, then check immediately and treat with a low treatment).

Food to be enjoyed:

____

Carbohydrates to be consumed per research:

____

Time of fast acting insulin dose:

____

Time of first bite of delicious food:

____

30 minutes after first bite:

____

60 minutes after first bite:

____

2 hours after first bite:

____

4 hours after first bite:

____

GREAT job! Now you know if your fast acting insulin dose needs adjusted for this food. Ask your Endocrine team if you need more help. Go forth and conquer all the yumminess!

The Emotional and Mental Side of Diabetes – Stress, Burnout, and Being Human

Let's face it: Type 1 Diabetes isn't just a physical condition—it's an emotional and mental marathon. Between carb counting, alarms going off at any hour of the night, and the never-ending unpredictability of blood sugars, it's normal to feel overwhelmed sometimes. And that's okay. In this chapter, we'll explore how to care for your mental health while living with T1D, because your brain deserves just as much attention as your pancreas.

1. It's Okay to Feel All the Feelings

Living with T1D can stir up a cocktail of emotions: frustration, fear, guilt, or even burnout. You're not alone, and these feelings don't mean you're failing. They mean you're human.

Common Emotional Challenges with T1D:

- **Burnout:** Constantly managing diabetes can feel exhausting.
- **Fear of Lows/Highs:** Worrying about extreme blood sugar swings can create anxiety.
- **Guilt:** Feeling bad about eating certain foods or seeing "bad" numbers.
- **Isolation:** Feeling like no one understands what you're going through.

2. Managing Stress: The Blood Sugar Bully

Stress doesn't just mess with your head; it messes with your blood sugar too. Stress hormones like cortisol can cause unexpected highs, leaving you feeling even more frazzled.

How to Tackle Stress:

- **Breathe:** Deep breathing or meditation can calm your mind and your blood sugar. Try apps like Calm or Headspace to guide you.
- **Move Your Body:** Exercise is a great stressbuster, whether it's a walk, yoga, or dancing like no one's watching.
- **Journal:** Write down what's bugging you. Getting it out of your head can make it feel more manageable.
- **Talk About It:** Share your feelings with someone you trust—a friend, family member, or therapist.

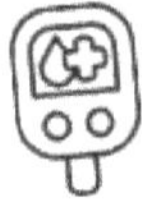

Take notes and consider journaling to help learn how stress affects your blood sugar, and keep notes about what works for YOU to lower your stress.

3. Coping with Diabetes Burnout

What is Diabetes Burnout?

It's when you're tired of thinking about T1D every second of the day. You might feel like ignoring blood sugars, skipping boluses, or avoiding diabetes altogether.

How to Manage Burnout:

- **Take Small Steps:** Start with one thing, like checking the carb app once a day. Small wins build momentum.
- **Give Yourself Grace:** Nobody gets it perfect all the time. Forgive yourself for the hard days.
- **Talk to Someone:** Share your feelings with a friend, family member, or therapist. Sometimes just saying it out loud helps.

4. Building Emotional Resilience

Focus on What You Can Control

You can't control every blood sugar spike, but you can control how you respond. Treat yourself with kindness when things don't go as planned.

Create a Routine That Works for You

Routines can make T1D feel less overwhelming. Plan your meals, check-ins, and supplies to reduce decision fatigue.

Celebrate Small Wins

Did you treat a low before it got bad? Take your insulin before a meal? These are victories, and they deserve celebration!

5. Dealing with the “Numbers Game”

You Aren’t Your Numbers

Blood sugars are data, not a judgment of your worth. A high or low doesn’t make you a “bad diabetic.” It just means your diabetes plan needs an adjustment.

Reframe Your Perspective:

- Instead of: “Ugh, my blood sugar is 250—I failed.”
- Try: “My blood sugar is 250. I’ll correct it and move on.”

Resilience Tip: Aim for Progress, Not Perfection

“Perfect” control isn’t possible and chasing it will only drain you. Focus on steady improvement and giving yourself grace.

6. Finding Joy Amidst the Challenges

Rediscovering What Makes You Happy

Diabetes can feel all-consuming, so it’s important to nurture hobbies, passions, and activities that bring you joy.

- **Art or Music:** Creative outlets can help you process emotions.
- **Sports or Movement:** Exercise boosts your mood and helps with blood sugar management.

- **Spending Time with Loved Ones:** Connection is a powerful antidote to stress.

Practice Gratitude

Even on tough days, there's always something to appreciate. It could be a supportive friend, a delicious meal, or just making it through the day.

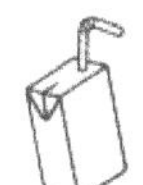

This might sound crazy to most of you, but I've always felt fortunate to have juvenile diabetes.

I was diagnosed in May of 1975—yes, over 50 years ago! My mom took me in for my 6-year-old checkup, and my blood sugars were elevated. We went for further testing at Egleston Children's Hospital in Atlanta, Georgia. I failed the tests and was admitted for a week. Honestly, it was harder for my family than it was for me. I remember being surrounded by children with severe physical and mental challenges. I was lucky—I could run, play, walk. All I had to do was take one shot a day.

7. When to Seek Help

Signs You Might Need Extra Support:

- Feeling overwhelmed more often than not.
- Struggling with anxiety, depression, or feelings of hopelessness.
- Avoiding diabetes care because it feels too hard.

Where to Turn:

- **Therapists:** Look for someone experienced with chronic illness or diabetes.
- **Your Care Team:** Don't be afraid to share your struggles with your doctor or diabetes team. They work with people every day who feel some of the same things!
- **Support Groups:** Connecting with others who "get it" can be incredibly validating. (Diabetes camps are a great way to connect!)

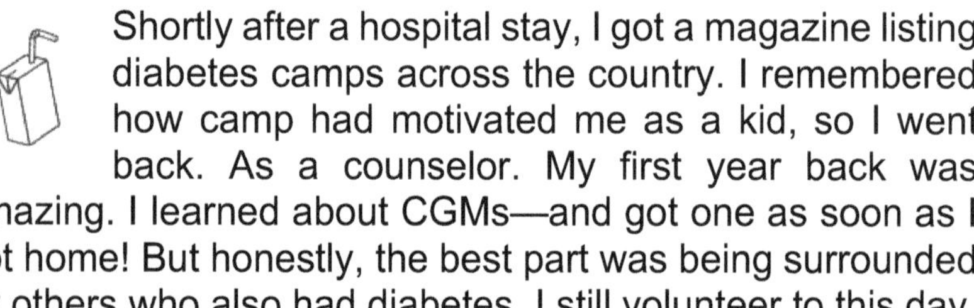

Shortly after a hospital stay, I got a magazine listing diabetes camps across the country. I remembered how camp had motivated me as a kid, so I went back. As a counselor. My first year back was amazing. I learned about CGMs—and got one as soon as I got home! But honestly, the best part was being surrounded by others who also had diabetes. I still volunteer to this day.

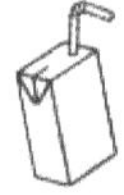 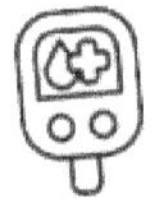 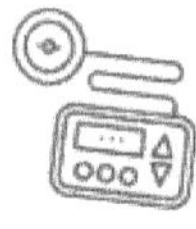 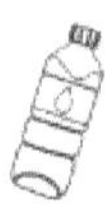 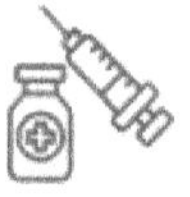

PRO TIP: You're Not Alone

It's easy to feel isolated with T1D, but there's a whole community out there that understands. Whether it's online forums, local meetups, or a diabetes camp, finding your tribe can make all the difference.

Living with T1D is a marathon, not a sprint. Some days will be harder than others, but with resilience, self-compassion, and the right support, you can thrive.

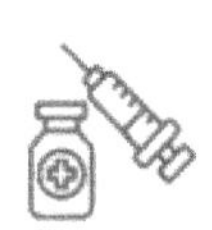

ACTIVITY: If you are feeling alone right now with your T1D, pull up your favorite social media app. Search 'T1D' or 'Type 1 Diabetes' and see what comes up. Prepare to be surprised! The #DOC (Diabetes Online Community) is large and strong!

Staying Active with T1D – Exercise, Sports, and Activity

Whether you're running marathons, hiking mountains, doing yoga or walking the dog, staying active is a fantastic way to keep your body healthy and your mind happy. Exercise can help with blood sugar management—but it also adds some twists to the diabetes game. Don't worry; with the right tools and mindset, you can handle it all.

Why Exercise Affects Blood Sugar

Exercise makes your muscles more sensitive to insulin, which can cause your blood sugar to drop during and after activity. But certain types of exercise (like weightlifting or sprints) can also trigger a short-term spike. It's like your blood sugar has its own workout routine.

Common Blood Sugar Responses:

- **Aerobic Exercise (e.g., running, cycling):** Tends to lower blood sugar.
- **Anaerobic Exercise (e.g., weightlifting, sprints):** May cause a short-term rise before leveling out.
- **Mixed Activities (e.g., sports, dancing):** Can create unpredictable blood sugar swings.

Knowing what to expect can help you plan ahead.

1. Preparing for Exercise: The Pre-Workout Checklist

Before you dive into your workout, take a few steps to set yourself up for success:

Check Your Blood Sugar:

- Aim for a starting range of about 120–180 mg/dL (check with your healthcare team for your ideal range).
- If you're low (<100 mg/dL), have a quick snack like a banana or glucose tabs.
- If you're high (>250 mg/dL), check for ketones and correct if needed before exercising. Drink water.

Pack Your Essentials:

- Fast-acting carbs (glucose tabs, a dextrose-based candy, or a drink such as Gatorade).
- Your meter or CGM (Continuous Glucose Monitor).
- Water (hydration is key!).

Adjust Insulin if Needed:

- If you're using a pump, consider a temporary basal, or activity, rate. You may need to do this well before you start your physical activity.
- If you're on injections, talk to your doctor about adjusting your doses for exercise.

2. During Exercise: Stay in the Zone

Keep an Eye on Your Numbers:

If you're using a CGM, check periodically to make sure you're staying in range. If you don't have a CGM, take breaks to test with your meter.

Respond to Changes Quickly:

- If you feel low, stop and treat it immediately with 15–20 grams of fast digesting carbs.
- If you start feeling sluggish or your numbers are creeping up, take a break and re-evaluate.

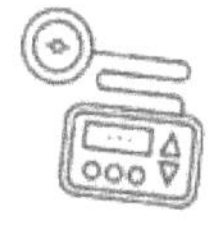

Some things that I learned that might be helpful and/or encouraging to you is that cold weather and exercise can make your blood sugar go down! My family has a hill behind our house so we sled and with the combination of the cold and sledding my blood sugar will tank. So, if you drink about a half a cup of juice, it will help you! Stress, anxiety, hormones, and sickness can make your blood sugar go up. There are many ways for you to get it down but I would recommend just taking a deep breath and then figure it out.

3. After Exercise: Post-Workout Blood Sugar Care

Watch for Delayed Lows:

Your body continues to burn glucose after exercise, which can lead to lows hours later (hello, 2 a.m. surprises). To prevent this:

- Have a snack with protein and carbs after working out.
- Check your blood sugar before bed if you exercise late in the day.

Hydrate and Refuel:

Drink water and eat a balanced meal to help your body recover.

4. Managing Sports and Adventure Activities

If you're into team sports, outdoor adventures, or competitive events, diabetes doesn't have to hold you back. Here's how to tackle bigger activities with confidence:

Team Sports:

- Let your coach and teammates know about your diabetes.
- Keep your supplies nearby during games and practices.
- Take breaks as needed—your health first.

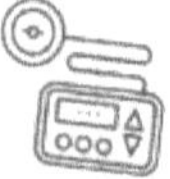

Sports are another obstacle in diabetes. Your blood sugar will react differently to every sport. The first few weeks of practice is learning how to regulate your blood sugar. I always put my Gatorade or a fast-acting snack next to the water and I'll sit out if I start to feel it going low. Another important thing is you *have* to tell your coach and possibly a few teammates. They need to know. Just remember your diabetes doesn't determine if you can or can't play sports or anything you love to do.

Hiking and Camping:

- Pack extra supplies (think twice as many as you think you'll need).
- Keep snacks and fast-acting carbs within reach.
- Test often, especially during long hikes.

Competitive Events:

- Practice your diabetes routine during training so you know what works.
- Stay calm under pressure—having a plan for highs or lows can ease your mind.

5. Finding Your Favorite Activities

The best exercise is the kind you enjoy. Don't force yourself to run if you hate running. Try different things until you find your groove:

- Love the outdoors? Go hiking, biking, or kayaking.
- Want something social? Try group fitness classes, dance, or team sports.
- Prefer solo activities? Yoga, swimming, or weightlifting might be your jam.

6. Staying Safe While Staying Active

Listen to Your Body:

If you feel off—low, high, or just "not right"—pause and check in with yourself. It's better to take a break than push through and risk feeling worse.

Have a Plan B:

Sometimes your blood sugar doesn't cooperate, and that's okay. Adjust as needed and try again another day.

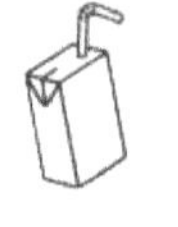

My mom made sure I stayed active. I played soccer, went to day camps and sleepaway camps with other kids who had diabetes. I still play hard and volunteer at camps today.

PRO TIP: Celebrate Every Step

Exercise with Type 1 Diabetes takes planning, but every step you take (literally and figuratively) is a win. Whether you're walking around the block or climbing a mountain, you're showing yourself and the world – and yourself - what you're capable of.

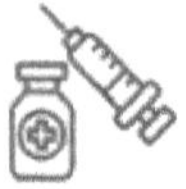

ACTIVITY: Pull out your phone (go ahead!) and search: "Olympic Athletes with Type1 Diabetes". Who knew!?

Traveling with T1D – Planes, Trains, and Blood Sugar Gains

The world is big, beautiful, and ready for you to explore. And yes, Type 1 Diabetes can come along for the ride! Traveling with T1D can feel like you're preparing for a NASA mission, but it's absolutely worth it. But don't worry, with the right preparation, you can explore the world (or just the next state over) without leaving your blood sugar behind. This section will help you navigate new destinations with confidence, curiosity, and a solid stash of glucose tabs – and prove there's nowhere you can't go!

Pre-Travel Prep

Before you hit the road (or skies), preparation is key. Here's how to set yourself up for a smooth adventure:

1. **Pack Smart (and Overpack a Little):**

   - Bring *at least double* the supplies you'd normally need for the duration of your trip.
   - Include insulin, test strips, CGM sensors, pump supplies, syringes/pens, glucose tabs, snacks, and batteries/chargers.

PRO TIP: Split your supplies between your carry-on and your personal item, just in case one bag goes missing. Never check your diabetes supplies. They can get lost, damaged, or freeze, which can ruin your insulin. Airlines MUST allow you a carry-on medical bag in addition to the usual carry-on allowance.

- Use the *Travel Checklist* at the end of this chapter to create your personalized packing list!

2. **Carry a Doctor's Note:**

   - A simple note explaining your T1D, medications, and devices can smooth things out with airport security or customs officials.

3. **Know the Local Resources:**

   - Research pharmacies, hospitals, and emergency numbers in your destination.
   - If traveling internationally, learn a few phrases like "I have Type 1 Diabetes" or "I need sugar" in the local language.

4. **Check Time Zones:**

   - Crossing time zones? Adjust your insulin schedule gradually to match your new routine.

Airports and Security

Airports can be stressful, but with a bit of know-how, you can breeze through TSA and beyond:

1. **Declare Your Supplies:**

- Let TSA agents know you have medical supplies. Most agents are familiar with them, but it doesn't hurt to give them a heads-up.
- Insulin pumps and CGMs shouldn't go through x-ray scanners—request a hand check instead.

Strange but true: They will dust your pump and your hands for explosive residue right after you walk through the scanner or get hand checked. Not joking. It's quick and easy – but allow yourself some extra time to get through security.

2. **Stay Cool (Literally):**

    - Use an insulated bag or Frio pack to keep insulin at a safe temperature during your travels.

3. **Keep Snacks Handy:**

    - Low blood sugar in the air? Airlines don't always have quick carb options. Pack glucose tabs, granola bars, or juice boxes in your carry-on.

4. **Opt for a pat-down:**

    - If you're uncomfortable with body scanners, you can request a manual inspection.

Eating on the Road

Different foods, strange schedules, and restaurant menus can throw off your routine. But there's always a way to manage:

- **Learn to estimate carbs.** Apps like MyFitnessPal or Carb Manager can help when you're faced with an unfamiliar dish.
- **Snack smart.** Keep low-carb snacks like nuts or cheese sticks on hand to avoid big spikes between meals.
- **Hydrate.** Dehydration can mess with blood sugar levels, so drink water often.

Time Zones and Insulin Dosing

Crossing time zones? Your insulin schedule might need adjusting:

- For **long flights**, stick to your home time zone until you land.
- For **extended trips**, gradually shift your insulin schedule by an hour or two each day leading up to your travel.
- If in doubt, consult your endocrinologist ahead of time to create a travel-specific plan.

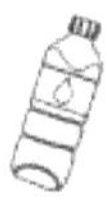

PRO TIP: Travel disrupts routines—that's part of the adventure. If your blood sugar isn't perfect, don't stress. It's all about staying as close to stable as possible and enjoying the journey.

Thriving in New Places

Exploring a new city, hiking in the mountains, or lounging on a beach? Here's how to keep T1D in check while soaking up the adventure:

1. **Adjust for Activity:**
   - Increased activity (like walking tours or swimming) may lower your blood sugar, so be proactive with monitoring, adjusting, and snacking.
2. **Mind the Climate:**
   - Hot weather can affect insulin absorption, while cold weather may make your hands too numb to test blood sugar. Plan accordingly!
3. **Try New Foods (Smartly):**
   - Sampling local cuisine is one of the best parts of travel. Just guesstimate carb counts as best you can, check your glucose often, and enjoy the experience.

Managing Highs and Lows on the Go

Traveling can throw curveballs at your blood sugar, but a little flexibility goes a long way:

1. **Lows Happen:**

- Always carry fast-acting carbs, no matter where you are. If you're hiking or exploring remote areas, pack extra.
- Example: "That Eiffel Tower view can wait—my glucose tabs are the real VIP right now."

2. **Highs Happen Too:**

- Dehydration is common while traveling, which can worsen highs. Drink plenty of water, adjust insulin as needed, and take breaks if you're feeling sluggish.

Long-Term Travel Tips

If you're traveling for an extended period, add these to your checklist:

1. **Refills Abroad:**

- Research how to refill prescriptions in your destination country. Some places require a doctor's note or local prescriptions.

2. **Stay Connected:**

- Use apps like Glooko or Tidepool to share your blood sugar data with your healthcare team, even from afar.

3. **Lean on the Community:**
    - Join local T1D groups or forums to connect with others and get insider tips.

Embrace the Journey

Traveling with T1D doesn't have to be daunting. Yes, it takes extra prep, but you're already a pro at managing the unexpected. The world is full of new foods, places, and people—and your T1D shouldn't stop you from experiencing them. Each trip teaches you something new about your resilience, adaptability, and ability to handle anything that comes your way.

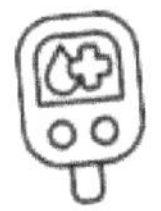

Traveling with Type 1 Diabetes has taught me responsibility and planning. Before trips, I pack extra supplies, insulin, insulin pumps, continuous glucose sensors, and snacks to treat my low sugars. I find ways to keep my insulin cold while traveling and refrigerate it as soon as I arrive. I've learned that changes in routine like travel, starting school, or beginning summer break can cause unexpected highs or lows, so I pay extra attention during those times.

Live in the Moment

Travel is about creating memories. Whether you're exploring new cities or relaxing on the beach, remember to enjoy yourself. T1D is part of your journey, but it's not the whole story.

Bon Voyage!

Wherever you go, your T1D doesn't have to hold you back. With the right preparation and mindset, you can turn any trip into an unforgettable experience. So grab your supplies, charge your devices, and set off on your next adventure—T1D and all. The world is waiting for you, and it's yours to explore.

Let's go, globetrotter! Your next adventure awaits.

PRO TIP: Go With the Flow
Travel days rarely go perfectly. Delays, missed meals, or unexpected activity levels can affect your blood sugar, but staying adaptable is part of the adventure.

BONUS PRO TIP: Take photos, journal your experiences, and celebrate every step of your journey. Whether it's a weekend getaway or a bucket-list destination, you're proving that life with T1D has no limits.

Extra Bonus Pro Tip: Wear medical ID jewelry, especially when traveling solo. It's a simple way to alert others to your condition in case of an emergency.

OK wait – one more Pro Tip: Don't be afraid to speak up about your needs. Whether it's at security or on a plan, most people are accommodating once they understand the situation.

ACTIVITY: YOUR T1D TRAVEL CHECK LIST

Let's start with the essentials. Packing for a trip with T1D means making sure you have everything you need for diabetes management. Here's your ultimate checklist:

- **Insulin:** Always pack extra. (Double what you think you'll need!)
- **Syringes, pens, or pump supplies:** Bring backups, and then bring backups for the backups.
- **CGM sensors or test strips:** Don't get caught without them.
- **Glucose tablets and snacks:** Hypo emergencies don't take holidays.
- **Glucagon and Ketone Strips:** Travel means unexpected glucose changes may occur. Be prepared in case of emergency.
- **Doctor's note:** Some airports or venues might require documentation for medical supplies.
- **Cooling packs:** Essential for keeping your insulin at a safe temperature.
- **Portable charger:** Because dead devices can't save your life.
- **Anti-nausea medicine:** Preventing or stopping vomiting quicky can help prevent significant dehydration, which could require an emergency visit.

- ____
  ____
- ____
  ____

- ○ ____

Talking T1D – Friends, Family, and Those Awkward Questions

Talking about Type 1 Diabetes can feel tricky. Sometimes it's a quick "Oh, I've got this!" and other times it's navigating well-meaning but clueless comments like, "So, you can't have sugar, right?" (Cue the inner eye roll.) Let's break down how to talk about diabetes with confidence, humor, and just the right amount of patience.

Why Talking About Diabetes Matters

Whether you like it or not, diabetes is a part of your life, and people are going to have questions. Opening up can:

- Help others understand your needs.
- Build a support system.
- Bust myths and educate people about what Type 1 Diabetes actually is.

But here's the thing: you get to decide how much you share and with whom.

1. Talking to Family: The Support Squad

Your family is often your first line of support—but they might not always get it right. They might hover, ask too many questions, or offer unsolicited advice. (Thanks, Mom, but I know how to count carbs!)

How to Navigate Family Conversations:

- **Educate Them:** Teach them the basics about Type 1 Diabetes, like how it's managed and what to do in an emergency.
- **Set Boundaries:** If someone's being overbearing, gently remind them you've got it under control. ("Thanks for caring, but I've been doing this a while now!")
- **Ask for Specific Help:** Whether it's grabbing juice for a low or understanding why you need to pause an activity to check your sugar, let them know how they can support you.

2. Talking to Friends: The Inner Circle

Good friends want to support you, but they might not know how. They also might not realize that joking about your pump being a pager from the '90s isn't actually funny.

How to Keep It Real with Friends:

- **Keep It Simple:** Start with the basics. "I have Type 1 Diabetes, which means my pancreas doesn't make insulin. I use insulin and carb counting to keep my blood sugar in range."
- **Answer Questions (If You Want To):** Some friends will be curious, and that's okay. Answer what you're comfortable with and redirect what you're not.
- **Speak Up:** If your blood sugar is low and you need a snack break or feel off, let them know. True friends won't mind pausing to help.

3. Talking to Strangers: The Curious Bystanders

Sometimes strangers get nosy. Whether it's the cashier eyeing your candy purchase or someone asking, "What's that stuck to your arm?" you've got a few options:

Your Toolkit for Stranger Encounters:

- **Educate:** "Actually, with Type 1 Diabetes, I can eat anything as long as I manage it with insulin."
- **Use Humor:** "Yes, I can eat that—and no, it won't explode my pancreas!"
- **Deflect:** "It's a medical thing. Don't worry, I've got it covered."

Remember, you're not obligated to explain your life to anyone. Share what you're comfortable with and move on.

4. Tackling Awkward or Rude Comments

Unfortunately, not everyone is tactful. Here are some common awkward comments and how to handle them:

Comment: "Did you get diabetes because you ate too much sugar?"

- **Educate:** "Actually, Type 1 Diabetes is an autoimmune condition. It has nothing to do with what I ate."
- **Humor:** "Nope! But I'd be rich if I had a dollar for every time someone asked me that."

Comment: "You're so brave!"

- **Gracious:** "Thanks! It's just part of my life, but I appreciate your kind words."
- **Real:** "I'm just doing what I need to do to stay healthy—like anyone would."

Comment: "Should you be eating that?"

- **Firm:** "I appreciate your concern, but I've got this under control."
- **Funny:** "Should you be asking that?"

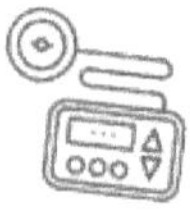

My biggest pet peeve with diabetes is when people ask me "Can you eat that??" The answer is yes. As long as you are responsible and dose for it, you can. I just respectfully respond with "The only thing I can't have is poison." You should see their faces!

5. Talking to Teachers, Coaches, or Employers

Sometimes you need to talk about diabetes in a professional or school setting. These conversations can feel intimidating, but they're important to ensure your needs are met.

What to Share:

- **The Basics:** Let them know you have Type 1 Diabetes and might need breaks to check your blood sugar, eat, or take insulin.
- **Emergency Plans:** Explain what to do if you have a low or high blood sugar.

- **Specific Requests:** For example, keeping snacks on hand during practice or flexibility with deadlines if you're feeling unwell.

Advocating for yourself is a skill—and the more you do it, the easier it gets.

Talking about diabetes is empowering because it puts you in charge of the story. Share what feels right, and don't worry about the rest. You're not just educating people—you're showing them how strong and capable you are.

PRO TIP: Sometimes talking about our diabetes is renewing, and sometimes it's just simply draining! Be aware of your energy level, and remember it is absolutely a-OK to tell someone "Hey, can we talk about this another time?"

ACTIVITY: Is there someone you've been avoiding having The Diabetes Talk with? Jot down some notes about what you want to say. Having the words written down can make it easier when the time comes to have the conversation:

____

____

____

____

____

____

____

____

____

Thriving at School, Work, and Beyond – Advocating for Yourself with T1D

Life doesn't pause for Type 1 Diabetes, and whether you're sitting in a classroom, clocking in at work, or chasing your dreams elsewhere, managing T1D in these spaces can feel like juggling flaming swords. The good news? You've got this. Advocacy, preparation, and a touch of humor go a long way. Let's dive into navigating school, work, and the rest of life like the T1D pro you are.

1. Owning Your T1D in School

Why Advocating Matters

School can be stressful enough without worrying about lows during algebra or explaining your pump in gym class. Advocating for your needs helps you stay safe and focused.

Set Up a Plan:

- **504 Plan (U.S. Schools):** This legally protects your rights and accommodations, like extra time for tests, access to snacks, or breaks to check blood sugar.
- Your 504 Plan can accompany you to college. You will work with your schools Disabilities Services to formulate your own plan.

- **Talk to Teachers:** Most teachers want to help but might not know how. A quick conversation about your needs can make a big difference.

What to Keep in Your Backpack:

- Glucose tabs or snacks.
- Extra pump supplies, syringes, or pens.
- A meter and CGM reader.
- A water bottle (hydration is your friend).

Handle the Curious Questions:

- "What's that on your arm?"
- Your reply: "It's my CGM—it helps me keep my blood sugar in check. Pretty cool, right?"
- "Why do you get to eat during class?"
- Your reply: "My pancreas retired early, so I have to step in. Snacks keep me safe."

2. Crushing It at Work

Know Your Rights

- In the U.S., the Americans with Disabilities Act (ADA) protects you from discrimination and allows for reasonable accommodations.
- Reasonable accommodations might include a flexible break schedule, a private space to check blood sugar, or the ability to keep snacks at your desk.

Tips for a Smooth Workday:

- **Tell Your Boss (When You're Ready):** While you're not required to disclose your diabetes, letting your employer know can help them support you.
- **Create a Routine:** Keep your supplies organized, set alarms for blood sugar checks if needed, and plan meals or snacks to keep things steady.
- **Handle Meetings:** If you need to check your blood sugar or treat a low during a meeting, do it discreetly or let your team know ahead of time.

Thriving in High-Stress Jobs:

Stress can send blood sugars haywire. Build stress-reducing habits, like short walks, mindfulness exercises, or regular breaks to breathe and reset.

3: Navigating Social Life with Confidence

At parties, on dates, or hanging out with friends, T1D is just one part of you. Don't let it stop you from showing up and having fun.

Addressing Awkward Moments:

- **When You're Low:** Say: "I just need a minute to fix my blood sugar. Then I'll be good to go."
- **When People Ask Questions:** Most questions come from curiosity, not judgment. A simple, "This is my CGM/insulin pump—helps me stay healthy!" is often enough.

Dating with Diabetes:

- Be upfront when you feel ready.
- If someone doesn't get it or is judgmental, they're not your person.

4. Handling Emergencies Like a Boss

Prepare for the Unexpected:

- **Emergency Stash:** Keep backup supplies at school, work, or your car—think insulin, snacks, glucagon, ketone strips, and extra pump supplies.
- **Share Your Plan:** Make sure a few people (coworkers, friends, teachers) know how to recognize and respond to low or high blood sugar emergencies.

Build a Safety Network:

Having a support system—friends, coworkers, or classmates who understand T1D—can make a huge difference.

5. Advocating for Yourself

Speak Up When You Need To:

- At school or work, advocate for your needs calmly and confidently.
- Remember, you're not being "difficult"—you're taking care of your health.

Educate Others (When You Feel Like It):

Sometimes, people just don't know what T1D entails. A quick explanation can dispel myths and make things easier for everyone.

Pick Your Battles:

Not every comment or question deserves your energy. Choose when to educate and when to let it roll off your back.

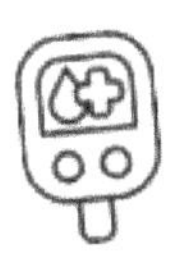

Diabetes has also taught me how important it is to advocate for myself. If a pump or glucose monitor fails, I call it in to get replacements. If my blood sugar won't come down despite insulin on board, I know how to troubleshoot by using a pen correction, changing a pump, or switching to a different vial of insulin if needed. These skills didn't come naturally or overnight, but they've made me more confident and independent.

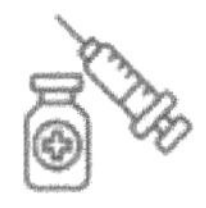

My mom taught me self-advocacy early. She trained teachers, coaches, babysitters—anyone who needed to know. When kids complained that I got "special snacks," and then their parents complained, we held a school assembly. I demonstrated glucose checks, injections, and explained highs and lows. No one complained again.

PRO REMINDER: You're More Than Diabetes

At school, work, and beyond, diabetes might shape some of your routines, but it doesn't define you. Your strengths, passions, and dreams are what matter most. You're not "the diabetic kid" or "the diabetic coworker." You're a rock star who happens to manage Type 1 Diabetes like a pro.

ACTIVITY: Did you know that positive visualization can help us to speak up for ourselves if we're feeling nervous, and help calm us down after having a conversation that was completely draining? The HearthMath Institute recommends this breathing and visualization activity, give it a try:

Close your eyes and focus on your heart, breathing a little bit deeper and slower than usual. Now, make a sincere attempt to experience a regenerative feeling such as appreciation or care. You can think about someone or something that you love, a fun activity, a pet, or just think about a happy memory.

Do this a few times if needed, it's a GREAT tool to have in your back pocket.

Love, Relationships, and T1D – Navigating the Feels

Relationships can be a wild ride: exciting, nerve-wracking, messy, and magical—all at once. T1D into the mix, and you've got an added layer of complexity. Whether you're dating, building friendships, or navigating long-term partnerships, T1D becomes a part of your journey. But don't worry—this chapter is here to help you rock your relationships with honesty, humor, and confidence.

Opening Up About T1D

The first step in any relationship is communication. But how do you bring up T1D without it feeling like a big deal? Here are some tips:

- **Be Honest:** Share your experience in a way that feels natural. You don't need to spill everything at once—just be real.
- Example: "By the way, I have Type 1 Diabetes. It just means I need to manage my blood sugar, but it doesn't stop me from doing anything I love."
- **Answer Questions:** Most people are curious, not judgmental. Be patient and open if they have questions—this can be a great way to educate them.
- **Set the Tone:** If you're confident and casual about your T1D, they'll take your lead.

Dating with T1D

Dating is already a mix of butterflies and nerves—add T1D, and you might feel even more anxious. But here's the thing: the right people will care about you, not your pancreas.

1. **First Date Basics:**

    - Pack your supplies discreetly but confidently—no need to hide them.
    - Mention T1D if it comes up naturally, like when you're ordering food or pulling out your meter.
    - Avoid overthinking it. If they're interested in you, T1D won't change that.

2. **Handling Awkward Moments:**

    - Blood sugar checks or pump beeps during a date? Laugh it off.
    - Example: "That's just my pancreas impersonator reminding me I'm alive."
    - Hypo during a date? It's okay to pause, treat, and explain.
    - Example: "I need to handle a quick low—can you be my glucose cheerleader?"

3. **Know Your Boundaries:**

    - If someone makes you feel weird or dismissive about T1D, that's on them—not you. Respect yourself enough to walk away from anyone who doesn't appreciate all of you.

Long-Term Relationships

When you're in a deeper relationship, T1D inevitably becomes part of the picture. Here's how to navigate the challenges while keeping the love strong:

1. **Educate Your Partner:**
    - Teach them the basics, like how to recognize and treat lows or what high blood sugar feels like.
    - Share your routines, like carb counting or pump management, so they understand your day-to-day.
2. **Involve Them (If You Want):**
    - Some people love being involved—helping with glucose tabs or learning how to calculate insulin.
    - Others might prefer to let you take the lead, and that's fine too. Communicate what works for you.
3. **Be Honest About Tough Days:**
    - If T1D is overwhelming, let your partner know. You don't have to hide your struggles.
    - Example: "Today's been a rough diabetes day. I could use some extra patience."

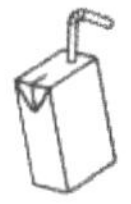

I'm so grateful for meeting my husband over 30 years ago. He's supported me through several severe high and low blood sugar levels. Make sure you find someone as supportive!

Friendships and Social Circles

T1D isn't just about romantic relationships—it's also part of how you connect with friends.

1. **Normalize It:**
   - Check your blood sugar, take your insulin, or treat lows around your friends. The more you normalize it, the more they will too.

2. **Teach Them the Basics:**
   - Close friends should know how to spot a low or where you keep your supplies.
   - Example: "If I'm acting weird or sluggish, just hand me some juice."

3. **Set Boundaries:**
   - If someone makes rude comments or jokes, address it directly but calmly.
   - Example: "I know you didn't mean harm, but jokes about diabetes aren't cool—they oversimplify a serious condition."

Love Yourself First

The most important relationship you'll ever have is with yourself. T1D can test your patience, resilience, and self-esteem, but it's also an opportunity to practice self-love.

1. **Celebrate Small Wins:**
    - Managed a tricky day? Give yourself credit.
    - Example: "I nailed my pre-bolus timing today. Go me!"

2. **Forgive Yourself:**
    - Blood sugars out of range? Forgot a bolus? You're human, not a robot. Learn and move forward.

3. **Focus on What You Love:**
    - T1D doesn't define you. Focus on your passions, hobbies, and relationships that bring you joy.

You Are More Than Your T1D

Your worth isn't tied to your blood sugar levels or how well you "manage" T1D. You're a whole, amazing person who happens to have a quirky pancreas.

Relationships Built to Last

Whether it's your best friend, your partner, or the most important relationship of all—your relationship with yourself—T1D is just one part of the puzzle. Open communication, honesty, and a little humor go a long way in strengthening those connections.

So, keep loving fiercely, laughing loudly, and living fully. The right people will see all of you—the struggles, the triumphs, and the unstoppable spirit that makes you who you are. And trust us, they'll love every bit of it.

PRO TIP: Do not keep your diabetes a secret from someone you want to have a relationship with (platonic or romantic). If someone is not interested in your diabetes, never asks questions, and isn't supportive when you need some extra help – they simply aren't for you. This doesn't mean they are a bad person, it just means they are not quite right for YOU.

ACTIVITY: Create a 30-second "T1D elevator pitch" so you're ready when the topic comes up. Something short, clear, and light-hearted does the trick. (An elevator pitch is a brief, confident explanation of your T1D that you could share in the time it takes to ride in an elevator).

____

____

____

____

____

____

____

____

____

____

____

____

Big Dreams, Bigger Goals – Chasing Your Ambitions with T1D

Type 1 Diabetes doesn't get to decide the size of your dreams. Whether you want to climb mountains, start your own business, or become the next Broadway star, your goals are still valid and achievable. T1D might add a few extra steps (and snacks) to the journey, but it doesn't mean you can't go the distance.

In this section, we'll talk about setting ambitious goals, tackling the challenges that come with them, and living life on your terms

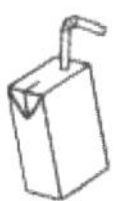

My first endocrinologist saw me from age 6 to 13. He told me I'd never have children and wouldn't live past 30. Well, I never had kids—but I'm well past 30. I sure showed him!!!

1. Dream Big, Plan Smart

Define Your Goals

Start by getting clear about what you want. Big or small, your goals matter. Write them down and be specific.

- Instead of: "I want to get fit."
- Try: "I want to run a 5K within six months."

Break It Down

Big goals can feel overwhelming, so break them into smaller, manageable steps.

Example: If your dream is to become a chef:

- Step 1: Research culinary schools.
- Step 2: Experiment with new recipes at home.
- Step 3: Find a mentor in the food industry.

2. Tackling T1D-Specific Challenges

Challenge 1: Planning Around Blood Sugars

Low blood sugars don't care about your deadlines, workouts, or creative bursts.

- **Solution:** Build flexibility into your plans. Always have a backup snack, and don't beat yourself up if you need to pause to handle a high or low.

Challenge 2: Energy Levels

T1D can drain your energy, especially if blood sugars are out of range.

- **Solution:** Listen to your body. Rest when needed and focus on small wins on tough days.

Challenge 3: Fear of the Unknown

Trying something new can be intimidating—what if your diabetes acts up?

- **Solution:** Prepare as much as possible. Pack extra supplies, inform someone you trust about your condition, and remind yourself you've handled plenty of challenges before.

3. Thriving in Physical Goals

Exercise Like a Pro

From running marathons to mastering yoga, physical activity is possible (and encouraged!) with T1D.

Tips for Active Goals:

- **Know Your Patterns:** Learn how your body responds to different types of exercise.
- Aerobic activities (running, swimming) might lower blood sugar.
- Anaerobic activities (weightlifting, sprints) can sometimes cause spikes.
- **Fuel Wisely:** Have fast-acting carbs nearby, and don't skip meals before workouts.
- **Adjust Insulin:** Talk to your doctor about adjusting insulin doses on active days.

Celebrate Small Wins:

Every step counts. Whether it's finishing a workout or learning how to adjust for exercise, progress is progress.

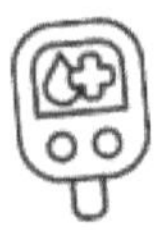

Dance is a huge part of who I am. It helps me express myself, manage stress, and feel confident and free in my body. Learning that diabetes would not take that away gave me hope during one of the hardest moments of my life: my diabetes diagnosis. Knowing I could still dance meant everything to me! Slowly, I began learning how to check my blood sugar, count carbs, give insulin, and listen to my body. At first, it felt overwhelming, but over time, it became part of my routine. I continue to dance, play sports, and chase my dreams!

4. Owning Your Professional Goals

Crush It in Your Career

T1D doesn't have to hold you back professionally. In fact, the skills you've developed—resilience, problem-solving, and time management—are assets in any career.

Pro Tips for Career Success:

- **Be Prepared:** Keep supplies and snacks at your workplace, so you're ready for anything.
- **Advocate for Yourself:** Don't hesitate to ask for accommodations if needed (like a private space for blood sugar checks).
- **Use Your Voice:** Share your story if you feel comfortable—it can inspire others and raise awareness.

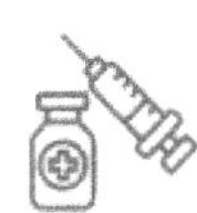

When I moved to a new city in my 20s, I had to take diabetes education classes before seeing an endocrinologist. A lightbulb went off: I could *be* a diabetes educator. If I had to live with this disease, I wanted to turn it into something positive. I became a Registered Nurse and later a Certified Diabetes Care and Education Specialist. Today, I help people around the world through classes, podcasts, webinars, and virtual visits. I love answering the questions people are embarrassed to ask, helping them build confidence, and supporting moms-to-be through healthy pregnancies.

Freelancing and Entrepreneurship

Dreaming of running your own business? Diabetes might mean extra planning, but the freedom to set your own schedule can be worth it.

5. Tackling Creative Goals

Express Yourself

Art, music, writing, acting—whatever your passion, diabetes doesn't have to hold you back.

Tips for Creative Pursuits:

- **Fuel Your Creativity:** Stay on top of your blood sugars during creative sessions so you can focus.
- **Incorporate T1D:** Some of the best art comes from personal experience. Let diabetes be part of your story if you want it to be.

- **Share Your Journey:** Your creativity might inspire others in the T1D community.

6. Staying Resilient When Life Gets Hard

When Progress Feels Slow

Everyone hits roadblocks. Blood sugars act up, life gets busy, or motivation wanes. That's normal.

Keep Perspective

Think of setbacks like detours, not dead ends. Adjust your approach and keep moving forward.

Build a Support System

Having people who believe in you—friends, family, mentors—can help you stay motivated. Don't be afraid to lean on them.

7. You Are Not Your Diagnosis

Remember: T1D is just one part of who you are. Your talents, dreams, and potential aren't defined by your blood sugar readings. You're capable of incredible things, and diabetes is just a part of your unique journey.

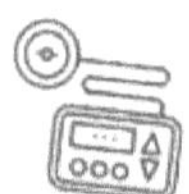

PRO TIP: Remember that the only person who gets to decide YOUR dreams and YOUR goals is...YOU! It isn't always easy, but don't let the negativity of others direct your path in YOUR life. You are UNSTOPPABLE!

ACTIVITY: What are some of your dreams and goals? You can do ANYTHING! Write them down here:

Sugar, Shots, and Substances – T1D in the Real World

Let's be real. By the time you hit your twenties, you might find yourself navigating new social situations: happy hours, parties, festivals, or chill nights with friends. For those with Type 1 Diabetes (T1D), these situations come with a unique set of challenges, especially when alcohol or recreational drugs are involved. This chapter is here to give you practical advice—without judgment—so you can have fun while keeping your health and safety in check.

Warning: adult content! No, not really. This is HUMAN content! This chapter has to do with the realities we face as we grow up with Betty. Are you ready? Nah, we never really are, and that is okay. Bear with me here as we review some adult-ish yet true content about growing up with diabetes.

The Lowdown on Alcohol

Drinking alcohol as someone with T1D isn't an automatic no, but it does come with risks. The big one? Alcohol can mess with your blood sugar levels. Here's how:

- **Hypoglycemia Risk:** Alcohol can suppress your liver's ability to release glucose, making lows harder to treat.
- **Delayed Lows:** You might feel fine while drinking, only to drop hours later—often while sleeping.

- **Carb Confusion:** Some drinks, like beer or cocktails, have lots of carbs, while others, like spirits, have none.

Tips for Drinking with T1D

1. **Eat Before You Drink:** Always have a solid meal with protein and carbs before drinking to stabilize your blood sugar.

2. **Pace Yourself:** Alternate alcoholic drinks with water to stay hydrated and keep tabs on how you're feeling.

3. **Know Your Drinks:**

    - **Beer:** Carbs galore! Be mindful of your intake, especially with craft beers.
    - **Cocktails:** Watch out for sugary mixers that can spike your blood sugar.
    - **Spirits (vodka, whiskey, tequila):** These are carb-free but can still cause delayed lows.

4. **Check Your Blood Sugar Often:** Before drinking, during, and especially before bed.

5. **Carry Supplies:** Always have glucose tabs or snacks handy.

6. **Tell Your Friends:** Let someone you trust know you have T1D and how to help in case of a low.

7. **Talk with your Diabetes Healthcare Team**: They will help you learn how to adjust your insulin plan safely if you decide to drink.

A Note on Recreational Drugs

Let's not sugarcoat this: recreational drugs come with risks, especially when you have T1D. They can affect your judgment, make blood sugar monitoring harder, and even mask the symptoms of highs or lows. That said, here's what you need to know:

1. **Marijuana (Weed):**

   - **The Good:** Weed generally doesn't directly affect blood sugar.
   - **The Risks:** Munchies (being very hungry after marijuana consumption) can lead to carb overload, and being "too relaxed" might mean you forget to bolus or ignore signs of a low.
   - **Pro Tip:** Bolus right as you start snacking, and set alarms to check your blood sugar.

2. **Stimulants (Cocaine, MDMA, etc.):**

   - **The Good:** Honestly, there's not much good here for people with T1D.
   - **The Risks:** Stimulants can spike your blood sugar (stress hormones) and mask low blood sugar symptoms, putting you at serious risk.

- **Pro Tip:** If you choose to use, have a trusted friend watch out for you and monitor your blood sugar closely.

3. **Psychedelics (LSD, Psilocybin, etc.):**

   - **The Good:** Minimal direct effect on blood sugar.
   - **The Risks:** Altered perception can make managing T1D confusing or overwhelming.

PRO TIP: Stick to a controlled environment and have a sober buddy who understands your T1D needs.

PRO TIP: **Alcohol + Drugs = Nope:** Combining substances increases the risk of dangerous blood sugar events that can lead to hospitalization…or worse. Just don't. STAY UNSTOPPABLE!

Socializing Without Substances

It's worth noting that you don't have to drink or use substances to have a great time. Being confident in your choice to abstain is just as cool. Try these alternatives:

- Mocktails or sparkling water with lime—they're festive and carb-friendly.
- Taking the lead on fun, sober activities like game nights, hiking trips, or creative group projects.
- Being the designated driver—you'll save lives and money.

Plan for the Morning After

If you do indulge, be prepared for the aftermath:

1. **Hydrate:** Water is your best friend.
2. **Check Early and Often:** Blood sugars can be unpredictable after a night out.
3. **Have a Backup Plan:** If you're not feeling great, give yourself grace and take the day slow.

Own Your Decisions

Life with T1D is a constant balancing act, and navigating alcohol or recreational drugs is no exception. The key is making informed choices that prioritize your health and safety without sacrificing your ability to enjoy life. You're not just surviving with T1D—you're thriving, and you deserve to live fully and fearlessly.

So, whether you're raising a toast with friends or sipping on a mocktail, remember: you've got this. Take care of your body, know your limits, and keep your blood sugar as steady as your confidence. Cheers to you!

PRO TIP: If you're wearing a Continuous Glucose Monitor (CGM), make sure your alarms are on and loud enough to wake you up.

ACTIVITY: Don't let peer pressure or social norms dictate your choices. Your health and comfort always come first. Let's use this space and time to create your 'What If' plan:

What if…I'm pressured to drink alcohol or use drugs?

____

____

____

____

What if…I'm not comfortable at a friend's house or party?

____

____

____

____

What if…I decided to try a little and things got out of control?

____

____

____

____

What if…after I participated, my blood sugars are out of control (low, high or both) and I can't get them managed?

____

____

____

____

The Power of Community – Finding Your T1D Team

Back to the club you didn't ask to join: this club has some of the most inspiring, supportive, and understanding people you'll ever meet. From sharing tips to swapping funny diabetes stories, finding your T1D community can make life with diabetes a whole lot easier—and more fun.

Let's explore how to connect with others, build a supportive network, and use the power of community to thrive.

1. Why Community Matters

You're Not Alone

It's easy to feel isolated with T1D, especially when no one around you understands why your phone alarm is going off for the fifth time today. A community of people who "get it" can remind you that you're not alone.

Shared Wisdom

Everyone manages T1D a little differently, and connecting with others is a great way to learn new tips, tricks, and hacks.

Emotional Support

Diabetes can be emotionally taxing, but knowing you have people who understand your struggles can help lighten the load.

2. Finding Your Circle

Online Communities

The internet is bursting with diabetes groups, forums, and social media pages where you can connect with others.

- **Facebook Groups:** Look for T1D-specific groups for advice, support, and camaraderie.
- **Instagram and TikTok:** Follow T1D influencers and hashtags like #Type1Diabetes or #DiabetesCommunity to find relatable content and people.
- **Reddit:** Subreddits like r/diabetes_t1 are filled with helpful discussions.

In-Person Connections

Sometimes, nothing beats face-to-face interactions.

- **Diabetes Camps:** These are a great way to connect with others, especially for teens and young adults.
- **Local Meetups:** Check if there are T1D support groups or events in your area.
- **Diabetes Conferences:** Events like Friends for Life or T1D summits are excellent for meeting people and learning more about managing T1D.

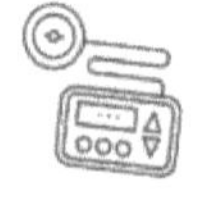

There are multiple places that have events for diabetics. There are camps, walks, and many more things. You can find one near you by doing an internet search. It helps to realize you aren't the only one in the world with diabetes.

Professional Support

- **Diabetes Care and Education Specialists:** They're a great resource for personalized advice.
- **Therapists:** Look for therapists experienced in chronic illness if you're seeking emotional support.

3. Sharing Your Story

Why Your Story Matters

Your experiences with T1D are unique, and sharing them can inspire and help others. You might even find that opening up strengthens your connections.

Ways to Share:

- **Social Media:** Post about your journey or join diabetes discussions online.
- **Blogs or Vlogs:** Create a space to share your experiences and tips.
- **Public Speaking:** Share your story at schools, events, or local meetups to raise awareness.

4. Giving and Receiving Support

How to Support Others

- **Be a Listener:** Sometimes, people just need to vent.
- **Share Tips and Resources:** If something works for you, let others know—it might help them too.

- **Celebrate Wins:** Whether it's an in-range A1C or surviving a rough week, cheer each other on.

Let Others Support You

It's okay to ask for help when you need it. Whether it's advice, emotional support, or just someone to commiserate with, leaning on others is a sign of strength.

5. The T1D Community's Superpower: Humor

The T1D community is hilarious. From memes about insulin prices to jokes about "diabetic-friendly" desserts, humor is one of the best ways to bond and cope.

Funny Things Only T1Ds Get:

- The eternal "pump tubing vs. door handle" battle.
- "Oh, your sugar is low? Have you tried not being diabetic?"
- When someone thinks your CGM is a nicotine patch.

Laughter really is the best medicine (next to insulin, of course).

6. Creating Your Own Community

Can't find a group that fits your vibe? Start your own!

- **Create a Social Media Group:** Invite others to join and share their stories.

- **Host Local Meetups:** Organize casual hangouts for people with T1D in your area.
- **Advocate for T1D Awareness:** Use your voice to make a difference in your community or beyond.

Living with T1D is hard, but you don't have to do it alone. By connecting with others, sharing your experiences, and building a supportive network, you'll find strength, inspiration, and maybe even lifelong friends.

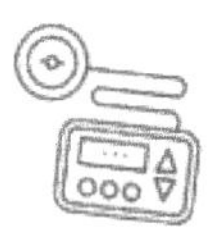

For me, the most important thing to remember about diabetes is that you *need* help. You can't do it alone. I've tried and failed. It just leads to diabetes burnout and you feel sick, tired, and you could even end up in the hospital. I would recommend finding someone who you trust and love to help you. You can talk to them and they can help you with your blood sugar and devices.

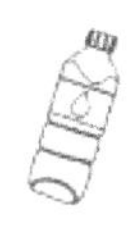

PRO TIP: Right now, you might not have much control over which endocrinology team you see. That's normal. But when you *do* get a say, choose the team that feels right for **you**. Not every provider is going to treat you like a partner in your own care—but you deserve one who does. Not every team is going to understand the chaos of blood sugar swings or let you talk honestly about your struggles without judgment—but you deserve one who will.

You need a team you can reach out to, feel comfortable with, and actually build a relationship with. And yes, that goal can be tough. Between insurance rules, long waitlists, and the giant ocean of endocrine options, finding the right match can feel like dating… but with more lab work.

Still, don't give up.

Advocate for yourself. Ask questions. Speak up when something doesn't feel right. You are allowed to want a team that listens, supports you, and helps you grow—not one that makes you dread appointments.

You deserve the best care and the best people in your corner. Keep going until you find them.

ACTIVITY: In one column, list the supporters and groups you have in your life that make your T1D easier. In the other column, list what you need to further support your journey:

HAVE	**NEED**

Advocacy 101 – Raising Your Voice for the T1D Community

Ready to change the world? You're in the right place. Advocacy is about using your voice and experiences to create change—whether it's raising awareness, fighting for better policies, or supporting others in the Type 1 Diabetes community. The truth is, no one knows T1D better than you. By speaking up, you can make a difference not only for yourself but for millions of others.

Why Advocacy Matters

Advocacy isn't just about making noise—it's about creating awareness and sparking change. Here's why it's essential:

- **Improved Policies:** Advocacy can lead to changes in laws and regulations, like better insurance coverage for diabetes supplies or increased funding for research.
- **Increased Awareness:** The more people understand T1D, the more empathy and support we can build in our communities.
- **Empowering the Community:** Sharing your story inspires others to speak up and advocate for themselves.

Telling Your Story to Support Advocacy

Your personal experience with T1D is your superpower. When you share your story to support advocacy, you make the challenges and triumphs of living with T1D real for others. Here's how to craft a compelling narrative:

1. **Be Authentic:** Speak from the heart about your journey.
2. **Focus on Key Points:** What do you want people to understand? Is it the financial burden of T1D, the emotional toll, or the need for accessible healthcare?
3. **Offer Solutions:** Highlight what changes could make life easier for the T1D community.

Advocacy in Action

So, how can you start advocating? Here are some ideas to make your voice heard:

1. **Social Media Advocacy**

    - Use platforms like Instagram, TikTok, and Twitter to share your story and educate others.
    - Join or create hashtags like #T1DStrong or #DiabetesAwareness to amplify your message.
    - Post about advocacy events or campaigns that others can support.

2. **Contact Your Representatives**

- Write letters or emails to your local, state, or national representatives.
- Share your experiences and ask them to support legislation that benefits the T1D community, such as insulin price caps or research funding.

3. **Participate in Awareness Events**

- Join walks, runs, or bike rides organized by diabetes organizations.
- Volunteer to speak at events or help with planning.
- Wear your T1D pride—shirts, bracelets, or pins can spark conversations.

4. **Collaborate with Organizations**

- Partner with groups like JDRF (Juvenile Diabetes Research Foundation), Beyond Type 1, or the American Diabetes Association.
- Volunteer your time or fundraise for their initiatives.

5. **Advocate in Your Community**

- Offer to speak at schools, workplaces, or local events to educate others about T1D.
- Work with local businesses to provide more T1D-friendly options, like carb-counting menus or hypo-friendly snacks.

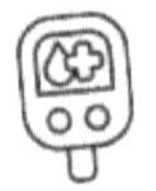

About a year after my diagnosis, I became a Youth Advocate with the Children's Diabetes Foundation. Becoming a Youth Advocate has been one of the most meaningful experiences of my life. It taught me that diabetes doesn't just affect one person—it affects families, communities, and millions of kids around the world. Being part of the foundation showed me that my story mattered and that I could use my voice to help others who were newly diagnosed or struggling. Through the Children's Diabetes Foundation, I've also been involved in fundraising efforts to help find a cure. I've participated in diabetes walks, traveled to Las Vegas for a golf tournament fundraiser, and even hosted my own craft fair to raise funds for diabetes research. These experiences showed me that even as a kid, I could make a difference. Diabetes may be part of my life, but it does not define who I am.

Fighting Stigma and Misconceptions

One of the biggest barriers the T1D community faces is misunderstanding. Many people still confuse Type 1 and Type 2 Diabetes or assume it's caused by poor lifestyle choices. Here's how you can combat stigma:

- **Educate:** Share accurate information whenever you hear misinformation.
- **Empathize:** Use kindness and patience when correcting others.
- **Normalize T1D:** Be open about your condition to show that people with T1D are living full, vibrant lives.

Advocating for Yourself

Advocating for others starts with advocating for yourself. Whether it's requesting workplace accommodations, asking for better care from your healthcare provider, or standing up for your needs in daily life, you deserve to be heard.

Your Voice Has Power

Never underestimate the impact of your voice. Speaking up for your needs is not selfish—it's necessary. You matter, and your advocacy sets an example for others to follow.

Dream Big, Act Bigger

The world needs advocates like you. Imagine what's possible if we all spoke up for affordable insulin, better education about T1D, and more support for the community. By working together, we can create a world where living with T1D is just a part of life—not the whole story.

So, what's your first step? Share your story, start a conversation, or join a movement. The world is listening, and change is waiting.

Ready to change the world, one voice at a time? Let's do it together.

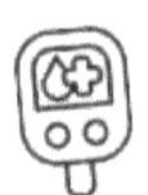

PRO TIP: One of the biggest lessons I've learned is that no two people with Type 1 Diabetes are the same. What works for me might not work for someone else. Our bodies react differently to food, hormones, stress, illness, and exercise. That's why it's important to keep learning, ask questions, and stay open to new tips and tricks that work for you, while setting personal boundaries when someone suggests something that you know isn't right for you or your T1D.

ACTIVITY: Get on the internet (yes, permission granted! Go ahead, do it right now!) and research what T1D events are going on in your community. Find one that looks interesting to you and add it to your calendar, even if it's months away! Make sure to chat with your grown-up if you need to arrange a ride or use a shared family calendar.

The Sweet Life – Thriving Beyond T1D

Hi! You've made it through this guide, and what a journey it's been! Living with Type 1 Diabetes isn't always easy, but it's teaching you strength, resilience, and how to roll with life's punches. This chapter is about looking forward—embracing your full potential, finding joy in the everyday, and reminding yourself that T1D is just one part of your incredible story. Let's recap everything we've covered in this adventure and journey book:

Redefining Success with T1D

Living successfully with T1D doesn't mean perfect blood sugars or always "getting it right." It means finding balance, making room for growth, and celebrating every win—big or small.

1. **Success Looks Different for Everyone:**
   - For some, it's learning to carb-count with confidence. For others, it's finally taking that dream trip or crushing a marathon.
2. **Celebrate Progress, Not Perfection:**
   - Remember: every day you show up for yourself, you're winning.
3. **Find What Fuels You:**

- Whether it's art, sports, writing, or advocacy, your passions and interests give your life purpose beyond T1D.

Building Your Resilience Toolbox

Over the course of this book, we've talked a lot about resilience. Now it's time to pull it all together:

1. **Community Connection:**

    - Surround yourself with people who "get it"—whether it's other T1D warriors or supportive friends and family.
    - Join online groups, attend meetups, or engage in advocacy work to feel part of something bigger.

2. **Mental Health Matters:**

    - Take care of your mind as much as your body. Therapy, mindfulness, and journaling are all great tools for managing stress.

3. **Self-Compassion:**

    - On tough days, remind yourself that you're human. T1D is complex, and you're doing the best you can.

Advocating for the T1D Community

Now that you've mastered your own journey, consider lending your voice to the broader T1D community:

- **Raise Awareness:** Share your story to educate others and fight stereotypes.
- **Advocate for Better Care:** Push for policies and advancements that make life easier for everyone with T1D.
- **Support Newbies:** Remember how overwhelming T1D felt in the beginning? Be the guide for someone just starting their journey.

A Reminder: You Are More Than T1D

I've said it before and I'll say it again because this is an extremely important message: T1D is part of your life—but it *doesn't define you*. You're a whole person with dreams, talents, and experiences that go far beyond blood sugar numbers.

Thriving, Not Just Surviving

This book isn't just about managing diabetes—it's about thriving. It's about finding freedom within the structure, joy amidst the challenges, and purpose in every moment.

You're not just someone living with T1D. You're a world-changer, an advocate, a friend, a dreamer, and a doer. You have everything it takes to live a full, adventurous, and meaningful life.

PRO TIP: Make a list of things that bring you joy and peace. When diabetes feels overwhelming, revisit this list:

____

____

____

____

ACTIVITY: Rewrite your narrative. Instead of thinking, “I’m stuck with this disease,” try, “I’m living boldly despite it.” The way you frame your journey matters.

YOUR T1D STORY

Write the Story Only *You* Can Tell

You've made it through this whole journey—learning, reflecting, rolling your eyes at diabetes, and maybe even surprising yourself along the way. Now it's time for something big: telling your own story.

Before you panic, take a breath. Your story doesn't have to be perfect, polished, dramatic, or written like a school assignment. It just has to be *yours*. The real version. The honest version. The version that sounds like you—not like what you think someone wants to hear.

When you write about your life with Type 1, don't feel like you have to sugarcoat the hard parts (pun absolutely intended). The tough moments matter. The funny ones matter. The confusing ones matter. Authenticity builds stronger connections than perfection ever will.

And here's the coolest part: Your story isn't set in stone. It grows as *you* grow. You can add to it, rewrite parts of it, or look back years from now and think, "Wow, I've come a long way." Even sharing a tiny piece of your story—a conversation with a friend, a moment with a teammate, a sentence you write here—can plant the seeds for change in someone else's life.

This is your space. Your voice. Your journey. Start wherever you want. Say whatever feels true. And remember: you're the only one who can tell this story.

Final Thoughts: Look How Far You've Come

Well, friends...did we do it? Did we conquer something big here?

Actually—yes. You did. You made it all the way through this guide (unless you're the kind of person who reads the last chapter first so nothing surprises you... in which case, welcome). Either way, you showed up. You stuck with it. That counts.

PRO TIP: It is time to CELEBRATE that you have finished this guide and journey book! Jump up and down and yell WAHOO! Do a dance, make a little move! Give yourself a high five and a hug – you are UNSTOPPABLE! (Remember how good this feels, celebrating, and make sure to CELEBRATE your T1D wins, even if they seem small).

ACTIVITY: Write down some words that describe how you are feeling about your diabetes right now:

____

____

____

____

____

____

____

Remember the words you wrote at the beginning of this journey describing how you felt about your T1D? Go take a look at them. GO ahead! Are some the same? Are some different? Have your perspective about your diabetes changed in any way? Write down your thoughts now:

____

____

____

____

____

____

____

____

____

____

Life with T1D will always have its ups and downs, but you've got the tools, the strength, and the heart to handle it all. So go out there and make the most of every single day. Laugh loud, dream big, and never forget: YOU ARE UNSTOPPABLE.

Thank you for letting this book be a part of your journey. Now, it's time to write the next chapter of your life—one filled with courage, joy, and endless possibilities.

Here's to the sweet life. Here's to being UNSTOPPABLE!

With love and hope,
One strong T1D warrior to another

Guest Voice Stories

Courtney's Story

I was diagnosed with Type 1 Diabetes in 1975, when I was six years old—yep, more than fifty years ago. My mom took me in for a routine checkup, and my blood sugar came back high. After more testing at Egleston Children's Hospital in Atlanta, I was admitted for a week. Honestly, it was harder on my family than on me. I remember looking around at kids with serious medical challenges and thinking, *I'm lucky. I can run. I can play. I just need a shot every day.*

In the early years, insulin didn't last very long. I'd take one shot, then two, and still spend half the day without insulin in my system. When I was fourteen, I switched to synthetic insulin and started bolusing for meals—six shots a day. Bolusing has always been tough for me, and it still is sometimes. We didn't have blood sugar meters yet, so we tested urine, which told us what my sugar had been hours earlier. It was almost always high. And yes, I wet the bed. A lot. If that happens to you, please know you're not alone.

My mom kept me active—soccer, day camps, sleepaway camps with other kids who had diabetes. That sense of community shaped me, and I still volunteer at camp today. When I was thirteen, I got my first glucometer. It took two minutes to give a reading, and the lancets felt like daggers. I ditched it for a while because I hated it.

I had a few scary moments growing up. On Halloween in 1977, I passed out from a low surrounded by candy. At nineteen, I thought I had the flu and cut back my insulin because I couldn't keep food down. I ended up in diabetic ketoacidosis with a blood sugar over 1800. I slipped into a coma for three days and spent a week in the hospital. That was my wake-up call.

In the early 1990s, I got my first insulin pump. It was life-changing—no more big injections, just a steady drip of insulin. Pumps back then were huge and had to be rewound and loaded manually, and yes, they could fail. In my forties, mine did. I became violently ill, ended up in the hospital for four days, and learned the hard way that you always need to know your doses and keep long-acting insulin on hand.

After that hospital stay, I went back to manual injections for a while. Around the same time, I found a magazine listing diabetes camps across the country. I remembered how much camp meant to me as a kid, so I went back—as a counselor. That first year changed everything. I learned about CGMs, got one immediately, and rediscovered the power of being surrounded by people who "get it."

Over the years, I've met people who've lived with diabetes for more than eighty years. I've built a life I love, found a partner who supports me through every high and low, and stayed connected to the diabetes community that helped raise me. I'm grateful for every educator, endocrinologist, and friend who never gave up on me.

I am one of you. And you are so fortunate to have the technology and tools available today. You can live a long, full, joyful life with Type 1 Diabetes. You can do anything. You can go anywhere. You can build a future you're proud of.

Stay healthy. Stay strong. Stay unstoppable!

Matti's Story

Hi! I'm Mattison, but everyone calls me Matti. I'm 15, a freshman in high school, and I live in Colorado Springs with my three younger siblings. I dance competitively, which basically means I spend half my life in a studio, covered in glitter, hairspray, or both. I started a podcast called "Sweet Talk with Matti". I also happen to have Type 1 Diabetes.

I was diagnosed when I was eleven, and nothing could have prepared me for how much my life would change. I was scared, confused, overwhelmed—you name it. I didn't know what Type 1 Diabetes even *was*, and I was terrified it would take away the thing I loved most: dance.

Before my diagnosis, I had never heard of T1D. I didn't understand how someone could need insulin just to stay alive or how blood sugar could affect every single part of your day. When I was admitted to Children's Hospital, everything felt huge and intimidating. New words. New rules. New routines. But the doctors, nurses, and counselors helped me understand that diabetes didn't mean the end of my normal life. They taught me what Type 1 is, how insulin works, and—most importantly—that I could still dance, play sports, and chase every dream I had.

Hearing that I could keep dancing meant everything. Dance is where I feel confident, expressive, and free. Knowing diabetes wouldn't take that away gave me hope during one of the hardest moments of my life. Slowly, I learned how to check my blood sugar, count carbs, give insulin, and listen to my body. It was overwhelming at first, but eventually it became part of my routine.

About a year after my diagnosis, I became a Youth Advocate with the Children's Diabetes Foundation. That experience changed me. It showed me that diabetes doesn't just affect one person—it affects families, communities, and millions of kids around the world. It taught me that my story matters and that I can use my voice to help others who are newly diagnosed or struggling.

Over the years, I've learned that managing T1D is about more than numbers. It's about balance, patience, and trusting yourself. I've picked up practical strategies that help me stay in range—like setting timers so I don't forget to eat, drinking extra water when I'm high, and being careful not to stack insulin. I've learned that technology is amazing, but not perfect. If my CGM says I'm fine but my body feels low, I trust my body and check with a meter.

Traveling with T1D has taught me responsibility and planning. I pack extra supplies, insulin, pump gear, sensors, and plenty of low snacks. I keep insulin cold on the road and pay extra attention when routines change—because travel, school schedules, and summer break can all make blood sugars act wild.

Diabetes has also taught me how to advocate for myself. If a pump or CGM fails, I call it in. If my blood sugar won't come down, I troubleshoot—pen corrections, pump changes, new insulin vials. These skills didn't come naturally, but they've made me more confident and independent.

One of the biggest lessons I've learned is that no two people with Type 1 are the same. What works for me might not work for someone else. Our bodies react differently to food, hormones, stress, illness, and exercise. That's why it's important to keep learning, ask questions, and stay open to new tips and tricks.

Through the Children's Diabetes Foundation, I've helped raise money for research—walks, fundraisers, even a craft fair I hosted myself. Those experiences showed me that even as a kid, I can make a difference.

Type 1 Diabetes doesn't control me, and it doesn't limit what I can achieve. If anything, it's made me stronger, more responsible, more compassionate, and more confident. I hope my story reminds other kids and teens with T1D that they're not alone—and that they can still dream big, work hard, and live full, happy, unstoppable lives.

Leah's Story

If you're reading this, you probably have diabetes or love someone who does. And if you're anything like me, you already know that diabetes can be really hard sometimes—but it also comes with moments of strength you never expected.

I was diagnosed about four and a half years ago, and the way it happened was… a lot. My family was hosting a Fourth of July party, and the whole day was a disaster. Someone threw a watering can at my head, my stomach hurt so badly I missed the fireworks, and I spent the entire night running to the bathroom. Everything I ate came back up, and even my stomach acid made an appearance. By morning, my mom took one look at me and said, “We’re going to the hospital.” We waited eight hours in the ER before they transferred me to Children’s Hospital. At midnight, I was admitted with no wait at all. A doctor told me I’d be going into surgery at 6 a.m. My appendix had burst, and I was really sick. I remember holding my stuffed elephant, Pudden, as they wheeled me into the operating room. The doctor put a mask on me and told me to count to ten. I only made it to three.

I spent almost the entire month of July in the hospital recovering. None of this had anything to do with diabetes—at least not at first. But because I hadn’t eaten in two weeks and was getting all my nutrition through an IV, the doctors checked my blood sugar. Even while fasting, it was in the 200s. They ran more tests, and that’s when I learned I had Type 1 Diabetes. I honestly thought it was something like the flu and that it would go away. Finding out it was forever was a lot to take in.

But slowly, you start to learn. You figure out how to take care of yourself, what works for your body, and what doesn’t. You build routines. You find your preferences. And you realize you’re stronger than you thought.

One of the biggest things diabetes has taught me is that you cannot do this alone. I’ve tried—and it only led to burnout, exhaustion, and feeling sick all the time. You need people. You need support. You need someone you trust who can help you talk through the hard moments, troubleshoot your devices, or just sit with you when you're frustrated. Asking for help isn't weakness. It's survival.

I also learned quickly that people will ask, "Can you have that?" My answer is always the same: "The only thing I can't have is poison." As long as I'm responsible and dose for it, I can eat what I want.

Finding community helps, too. There are camps, walks, and events for people with diabetes, and being around others who "get it" makes you feel less alone. My faith has also helped me. I'm not saying you have to believe what I believe, but trusting God has given me peace when things feel overwhelming. He's my anchor when diabetes feels like a storm.

I've picked up practical things along the way, too. Cold weather and exercise can make your blood sugar drop fast—sledding down the hill behind our house is basically a guaranteed low. Stress, anxiety, hormones, and sickness can make it go up. When that happens, I take a deep breath and figure out my next step.

There are good things about diabetes, too. You can get line-skip passes at amusement parks. You get to eat candy when you're low and no one can say anything about it. And the devices we have now—CGMs, pumps, all of it—make life so much easier. I keep extra supplies everywhere: in my sports bag, my suitcase, and my diabetes bag that goes everywhere with me. I even keep low snacks by my bed for nighttime lows.

Sports can be tricky with diabetes, but they're totally doable. Every sport affects blood sugar differently, so the first few weeks are all about learning. I keep Gatorade or fast-acting snacks by the water, and I always tell my coach and a couple teammates what to look out for. Diabetes doesn't get to decide whether I play or not.

Overall, diabetes has its highs and lows (pun fully intended). But there are people who will help you, and diabetes does not define who you are. You're still you—strong, capable, and unstoppable.

Tavia's Story

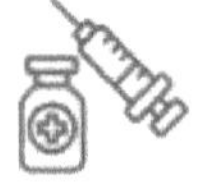

I was diagnosed with Type 1 Diabetes in April of 1981 when I was 2½ years old. A family friend noticed I kept asking for water and running straight to the bathroom, and I suddenly wanted naps I'd been refusing for weeks. She told my mom, "I think she has diabetes." My mom cried in the ER while waiting for the test results. I was admitted for a week so my parents could learn how to take care of me. They practiced injections on oranges, and my mom honestly thought I'd have to *eat* the oranges full of insulin before someone explained the shots were actually for me.

I don't remember being sick or scared. I remember one moment: standing next to my mom when a woman in a rocking chair rolled back and squished my big toe. We were all crowded into a hallway because a tornado-producing storm was passing through. That's my entire memory of diagnosis week.

Back then, families were sent home with urine tests because people thought finger pokes were too painful for little kids. My parents pushed for blood glucose strips and a lancet device nicknamed "The Guillotine." The strips were expensive and not covered by insurance, so they cut them into halves and thirds to make them last. You matched the strip color to the vial—20, 40, 80, 120, 180, 240, 400, 800—and waited a few minutes for a result. When glucose meters finally came out, my parents paid out of pocket. They were huge and took multiple steps, but they were life-changing.
I started on animal insulin—first cow, then pork. The needles were thick and long, and the injections left my thighs hard and scarred. Eventually, synthetic insulins and smaller needles made everything easier.

My mom taught me self-advocacy early. She trained teachers, coaches, babysitters—anyone who needed to know. When kids complained that I got "special snacks," and then their parents complained, we held a school assembly. I showed everyone how I checked my glucose and took injections, and we explained highs and lows. No one complained again.

Childhood lows were frequent and severe. Without CGMs and with older insulins, I had hallucinations and terrifying episodes. Today's insulins, pumps, and CGMs make lows so much more manageable, and I'm grateful every day for that progress.

I went to college before smartphones, before smart pumps, before any of the tech you have now. I used syringes and vials and carried a tiny notebook to calculate carb ratios and corrections. In my teens, I drifted from good management, but diabetes educators helped me relearn everything and take ownership of my care.

In my 20s, I had to take diabetes education classes before seeing an endocrinologist. During one class, a lightbulb went off: *I could be a diabetes educator.* If I had to live with this disease, I wanted to turn it into something positive. I went back to school, became a Registered Nurse, and eventually a Certified Diabetes Care and Education Specialist.

Today, I help people around the world through classes, podcasts, webinars, and virtual visits. I love answering the questions people are embarrassed to ask, helping them build confidence, and supporting moms-to-be through healthy pregnancies.

I have two teenagers now, and my oldest was diagnosed with T1D at 12. We screened through TrialNet and saw signs of developing diabetes ten years before his diagnosis. We participated in research studies because research is how better tools—and future cures—happen.

I'm grateful for every educator, endocrinologist, and supporter who never gave up on me. Diabetes takes a team. And if you don't have your team yet, keep looking. You're worth the effort it takes to find the right people. Remember: you are UNSTOPPABLE!

Thank You's!

PS – Hey, remember the part about community, and surrounding ourselves with supportive (and funny) people? It took an entire village to make this guide and journey book come to life:

Courtney: I would like to thank several people in my life for helping me stay alive #1 my Mom - Lorraine Woodman; #2 my endocrinologist for over 40 years - Doctor Chip Reed; #3 my new friend - Doctor Todd Alonso; and #4 especially my husband - Tim Dobbins.

Leah: Thank you to my family who has been by my side from day one, my staff at camp and my clinic who help me through the highs and lows (pun intended!), and my God who is my best friend in all of this!

Matti: I want to thank my mom for always being there for me and giving me so many opportunities that helped me become who I am. I know I'm not always the easiest teen, but I truly appreciate everything you've done and how you always find a way to support whatever I want to try. Thank you to my dad for cheering me on, helping me chase my goals, and being there through the hard moments. And thank you to my grandma, Aunt Missy, and Aunt Chaun for always supporting me, especially with my type 1 diabetes. It means so much knowing I have all of you in my corner. You all mean the world to me, and I'm so grateful for everything you've done. I love you so much.

Tavia: I would like to thank my parents, the Pediatric Endocrinology team and educators at the University of Iowa, Genesis Medical Center's Diabetes Educators, and the University of Colorado Hospitals Endocrinology, Diabetes, and Metabolism Clinic's Endocrinologists and Certified Diabetes Care and Education Specialists. I am who I am largely in part due to the ongoing education, advocacy, and support provided to me over the years. They never gave up on me (even when I pushed hard against counting carbs or trying an insulin pump!!). As they say, it takes a team. I'm so glad I've found mine!

www.ingramcontent.com/pod-product-compliance
Ingram Content Group UK Ltd.
Pitfield, Milton Keynes, MK11 3LW, UK
UKHW022003190726
13853UKWH00004B/1704

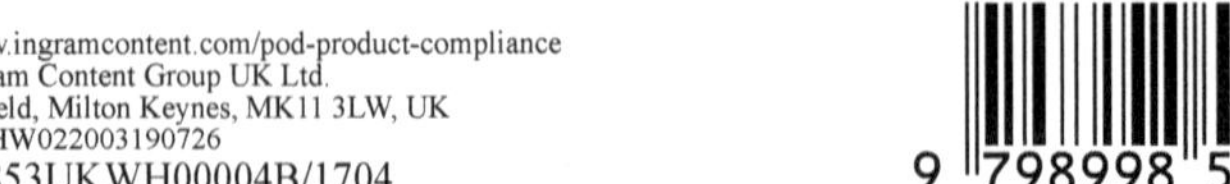

9 798998 541957